Sexual Health Promotion in General Practice

Sexual Health Promotion in General Practice

Edited by

Hilary Curtis
British Medical Association Foundation for AIDS
London

Tony Hoolaghan
Camden and Islington FHSA
London

and

Carey Jewitt
formerly with HIV Project

Published in association with
British Medical Association Foundation for AIDS
Camden and Islington Community Health Services NHS Trust
The HIV Project

Radcliffe Medical Press
Oxford and New York

Radcliffe Medical Press Ltd
18 Marcham Road, Abingdon, Oxon OX14 1AA, UK

Radcliffe Medical Press, Inc.
141 Fifth Avenue, New York, NY 10010, USA

Reprinted 1995
Reprinted 1996

British Library Cataloguing in Publication Data

A catalogue record for this book is available from the British Library.

ISBN 1 85775 131 0

Library of Congress Cataloging-in-Publication Data

Sexual health promotion in general practice / edited by Hilary Curtis,
      Tony Hoolaghan and Carey Jewitt. p.   cm.
    "Published ... in association with the British Medical Association AIDS Foundation."
    Includes bibliographical references and index.
    ISBN 1-85775-131-0
    1. Hygiene, Sexual—Study and teaching.   2. Family medicine.   3. Sexually transmitted diseases—Prevention.   4. Hygiene, Sexual—Study and teaching—Great Britain.   5. Family medicine—Great Britain.   6. Sexually transmitted diseases—Great Britain—Prevention.   I. Curtis, Hilary.   II. British Medical Association Foundation for AIDS.
    [DNLM: 1. Sex Behavior.   2. Family Practice—Great Britain.   3. Sex Education—Great Britain.   4. Health Promotion—Great Britain.   5. Sexually Transmitted Diseases—prevention & control—Great Britain.   HQ 58 S5187 1995]
    RA788.S4786 1995
    613.9'5—dc20
    DNLM/DLC
    for Library of Congress   95-22861 CIP

Typeset by Advance Typesetting Ltd, Oxfordshire
Printed and bound by Biddles Ltd, Guildford and King's Lynn.

Contents

About the contributors and editors

Dr Simon Barton is a consultant physician in HIV and GUM at Chelsea and Westminster Hospital. He wrote sections on talking about sex, including sexual history-taking (with Carey Jewitt). He is an MD and a Member of the Royal College of Obstetricians and Gynaecologists.

Simon Cavicchia is a lecturer in sexuality and sexual health at the National AIDS Counselling Training Unit, based at St Charles Hospital in West London. He has worked as a trainer and lecturer in sexuality and sexual health in a variety of settings, including as a training and development officer at the Family Planning Association, and undertakes consultancy work on developing integrated sexual health services and responses in GUM and primary care. He wrote sections on professional development and counselling approaches to health promotion and motivational skills (together with Brian Whitehead).

Dr Dílis Clare, who wrote the section on psychosexual problems, is a partner in a general practice in North East London, having qualified in the Republic of Ireland. She is a family planning instructing doctor, is training with the Institute of Psychosexual Medicine, and holds the Diploma of the Royal College of Obstetricians and Gynaecologists. Her interests include the development of primary care team-work, and she also undertakes disability equality training for health and social services.

Dr Elizabeth Claydon trained and worked as a GP in central Birmingham and is now consultant in GUM and HIV at St Mary's Hospital in Paddington, London. She wrote material on liaison between general practice, family planning and GUM services.

Hilary Curtis trained as a research chemist before becoming a policy researcher for the British Medical Association. She is now executive director of the BMA Foundation for AIDS, a charity that promotes education about HIV, AIDS and sexual health for professional groups and policy-makers. As well as editing and revising much of the text, she wrote about legal and ethical considerations (with Suzanne Smith).

Dr Chris Ford is a GP principal in Kilburn, North West London, and has a special interest in drugs and HIV. She wrote the section on the interactions between family planning methods and prevention of STDs and HIV, and provided much useful advice to the editors on the publication as a whole.

Kath Gillespie-Sells wrote the section on disabled people and sexual practice. She trained as a nurse, was a ward sister at Barnet General Hospital and lecturer in nursing, and spent eight years as head of training at the London Boroughs' Disability Resource Team. She is a counsellor, trainer, researcher and author, now working freelance and in a part-time post in welfare rights for disabled and elderly people. She is engaged in a national research project on disabled women funded by the King's Fund Institute, and is co-author of a book on the politics of disability and sexuality (published by Cassell in 1995).

Dr Lucia Grun is a part-time GP partner in North West London, and an MRC research fellow studying chlamydia with a view to screening in primary care. She has previously worked in GP collectives in Leyton and Hoxton, and as a research fellow in HIV in the Department of Primary Care at University College London Medical School. Her experience includes work for the Brook Advisory Centres and as a clinical assistant in GUM at University College Hospital. Her main contribution was to write material on targeting individuals at higher risk of HIV and STDs.

Sarah Hildyard wrote material reviewing research findings on sexual health and health promotion, for example on public understanding of safer sex messages. She qualified as a health psychologist and is currently at St Bartholomew's Hospital Medical College researching and designing sexual health promotion skills training for practice nurses in East London. She also lectures on psychology and communication skills and carries out freelance research and training in the field of sexual health and primary care.

Tony Hoolaghan is one of the editors and wrote the section on useful contact addresses. He is currently health promotion manager at Camden and Islington FHSA. His background is in psychology and research into primary care. He has worked in an academic department of primary care and was the researcher on the Health Promotion in General Practice project, which investigated the role of GPs in HIV prevention.

In addition to her role as one of the editors, Carey Jewitt wrote sections on sexual history-taking (together with Simon Barton), provision of condoms, and audit, monitoring and evaluation of services.

She is a researcher, and is currently working in London on a freelance basis, developing sexual health services for young men and in general practice. Her original background is as a trainer, but for the past five years her research interests have included family planning and sexual health issues in the general practice context, including sexual history-taking.

Mabli Jones trained as a nurse, and has worked as a ward sister in general medicine and HIV/AIDS and as a part-time practice nurse in a Well Woman clinic in Golders Green, London. She joined Barnet Family Health Services Authority as a primary care facilitator in 1993 and is now a nurse adviser there. She wrote material on the role of primary care facilitators.

Dr Elizabeth Murray is a job-sharing GP principal and a lecturer in the Department of Primary Health Care at University College London Medical School. She has previously worked as a clinical assistant in GUM at the Middlesex Hospital and wrote sections on the management of sexually transmitted diseases in general practice.

Dr Conamore Smith is a family planning doctor and is currently director of services for women at Parkside Health Trust, Raymede Clinic in West London. She wrote material on contraception provision, and on audit of family planning services.

Suzanne Smith is the project director of the HIV Integrated Health Care Project based at Hammersmith Hospital. She graduated in psychology and trained as a counsellor, and co-ordinated sexual health counselling services for primary care in San Francisco before moving to England. Her experience includes working as a senior health advisor in GUM and HIV services at Charing Cross and Westminster Hospital. She wrote much of the chapter on ethical considerations (jointly with Hilary Curtis).

Anita Weston wrote parts of the section on talking about sex, including material on partner notification and the language of sex, and material on attitudes to sex and sexuality. She is a registered general nurse, medical anthropologist and lecturer. Her background is in GUM nursing, and she has trained postgraduate nurses in sexually transmitted diseases nursing for the past five years. She is currently senior lecturer and subject quality co-ordinator in sexual health at the Centre for Sexual Health and HIV Studies, Wolfson School of Health Sciences at Thames Valley University, London.

Brian Whitehead's background is in training and counselling, including work as a counsellor in general practice. He now works as a lecturer and freelance consultant at East London and City Drug Services, having previously been senior trainer at the National AIDS

Counselling Training Unit. He wrote sections on professional development and counselling approaches to health promotion and motivational skills (with Simon Cavicchia).

Dr Henrietta Williams wrote much of the introductory material on aims of sexual health promotion, the general practice setting, roles of different members of the primary health care team, and opportunities for discussing sexual health. She is a principal in general practice at the Law Medical Group Practice, a large training practice in Wembley, Middlesex, and is GP fellow in HIV/AIDS and sexual health at Barnet Family Health Services Authority. Her experience includes working as a clinical assistant in GUM at the Central Middlesex Hospital, work in women's health and family planning at the Raymede Health Centre in West London, and in primary care medicine in Australia. She holds diplomas in child health and obstetrics and gynaecology and is a Member of the Royal College of General Practitioners and of the Faculty of Family Planning.

Foreword

Sex, sexual health, sexual health promotion, are all relatively new areas for us to think about in primary care. Issues pertaining to this emotive area of the human condition are common in general practice. However, they are often not addressed because of a lack of understanding, lack of training and fears concerning our own sexuality or the sexuality of others.

Sexual health is a vital component of our well-being; whether we are old or young, gay or heterosexual, disabled or able-bodied, black or white. The *Health of the Nation* document acknowledges the primacy of sexual health. It specifically recognizes that teenage pregnancy rates and rates of sexually transmitted diseases, of which HIV infection is one, are reflections of unmet community need. To be able to take on this challenge, clinicians need help in the form of up-to-date, accessible information as well as further training.

These are some of the reasons why we, as the Royal College of General Practitioners Working Party on HIV and AIDS, welcome this publication. It provides a sound theoretical base, with clear information to help us think about sexual health. It provides assistance on taking a sexual history, assessing risk in different people, recognizing needs in different groups, managing common problems and, most importantly, accessing extra help.

We hope that the whole range of professionals working in primary care will have access to this publication and will be able to use it in their work. We wish it every success.

On behalf of the AIDS
Working Party
Royal College of General Practitioners
August 1995

Editors' introductory note

This book is intended as a source of practical ideas and guidance for general practice teams who want to develop their role in enabling patients to adopt healthy, fulfilling and responsible patterns of sexual behaviour. We hope that every GP, practice nurse, receptionist, health visitor or other member of the primary care team will find something in this book that appeals to them and can be used in their routine practice.

However, no two general practices are alike. There are real differences between urban and rural areas, between practices serving populations with higher and lower prevalences of HIV and sexually transmitted diseases, and between the personal styles of different practitioners. As yet, no overall clinical protocol for sexual health promotion in general practice has been thoroughly evaluated and shown to be effective. Therefore, this book does not advocate a particular way of working as the 'gold standard' of good practice. Rather, it aims to provide a menu of options and ideas, some of which may suit relative beginners, while others are intended more for health professionals who are already experienced and committed to sexual health promotion work. If you find something in this book that you cannot adopt into your work, you may wish to think about *why* it seems inappropriate or irrelevant to your particular practice environment, and whether you can devise an alternative approach with which you feel more comfortable. Sexual health promotion is very much an evolving art, and we would be interested to know how you get on, and what you have found helpful or unhelpful in this book.

The text was written by a large number of different authors, who are listed at the start of the book. In order to avoid repetition and create a consistent style, their original work has been extensively edited and revised, so no individual author should be held accountable for any errors that may have appeared in a section attributed to him or her. The editors are responsible for the final version. We very much hope that you will enjoy reading the book and refer to it often.

Finally, we would like to thank the Joan Dawkins Fund and North Thames Regional Health Authority for their financial support, without which it would not have been possible to produce this book.

Hilary Curtis
Tony Hoolaghan
Carey Jewitt
August 1995

1

Sexual health promotion: why, where and when

Aims of sexual health promotion

Many GPs and nurses are increasingly committed to sexual health promotion. This reflects the growing emphasis on health promotion and disease prevention in primary health care: in one study more than 80% of GPs thought that health promotion should be incorporated into general consultations.[1] The central philosophy of general practice – the care of the whole patient and his or her family – implies inclusion of sexual health promotion at every opportunity. The Royal College of General Practitioners (RCGP) advises that family planning and sexual health services are 'an integral part of primary care', and that general practice should offer 'care and advice on a wide range of sexual matters... and promote safer sex to *all* patients'.

This is in agreement with the government's strategy for the *Health of the Nation* (1992), which identifies HIV/AIDS and sexual health as one of five key areas for improving the health of the population. For primary care, recommendations on how to achieve the *Health of the Nation* targets include training for all staff, developing practice policies on sexual health promotion, condom distribution and establishing 'shared care' guidelines for treatment of sexually transmitted diseases (STDs) and HIV.

The *Health of the Nation* is based largely on an 'illness' model of reducing morbidity and unwanted pregnancies, and encourages simple behavioural messages such as practising 'safer sex'. However, the World Health Organization gives a broader view through its definition of sexual health, which comprises:

- a capacity to enjoy and control sexual and reproductive behaviour in accordance with a social and personal ethic

- freedom from fear, shame, guilt, false beliefs and other psychological factors inhibiting sexual response and impairing sexual relationships

*   freedom from organic disorders, diseases and deficiencies that interfere with sexual and reproductive functions.

Within this, sexual health promotion includes any intervention that improves a patient's physical or psychological sexual well-being. It encompasses many tasks performed in primary care, for example contraception provision, cervical smears, safer sex advice, psycho-sexual counselling and other aspects of mental health care.

The *Health of the Nation* objectives for HIV/AIDS and sexual health

*   To reduce the incidence of HIV infection

*   To reduce the incidence of other STDs

*   To strengthen monitoring and surveillance

*   To provide effective services for diagnosis and treatment of HIV and other STDs

*   To reduce the number of unwanted pregnancies

*   To ensure the provision of effective family planning services for those people who want them

Specific targets to be used as markers of progress towards these objectives

*   To reduce the incidence of gonorrhoea among men and women aged 15–64 by at least 20% by the year 1995

*   To reduce the rate of conception among the under 16s by at least 50% by the year 2000

*   To reduce the percentage of injecting drug misusers who report sharing injecting equipment in the previous four weeks by at least 50% by the year 1997

The strategy for achieving the objectives relating to HIV/AIDS

- Prevention: encouraging behaviour change through aware-ness campaigns, community initiatives, education, improved infection control, and prevention and treatment services for drug users

- Monitoring, surveillance and research: improving under-standing of the epidemiology of HIV, its transmission, natural history, prevention and treatment

- Treatment, care and support: provision of co-ordinated diagnostic, treatment, care and support services for different groups of people with HIV/AIDS, according to need

- Social, legal and ethical issues: fostering a climate of under-standing and compassion, discouraging discrimination and safeguarding confidentiality

- International co-operation: full and continuing exchange of information between countries, and discouraging coercive and discriminatory measures.

Health of the Nation (1992)

What is safer sex? A simplistic view

Safer sex means choosing sexual practices that carry less risk of STDs, HIV or unwanted pregnancy. The aim for most people is to reduce risk to a level they consider acceptable, rather than to eliminate it altogether. There is a complication in that some practices that are unlikely to transmit HIV may still transmit other infections.

Safe/low risk
Dry kissing
Hugging
Massage
Body to body rubbing
Deep (French) kissing (safe for HIV, may be some risk of STDs)
Mutual masturbation
Voyeurism
Telephone sex
Sadomasochistic activity without bruising or bleeding
Sex toys that are used on only one person
Sex fantasy
Dressing up
Blue movies
Food play
Penetration with fingers, wearing latex protection (with the
    proviso that if this causes injury, it may increase the risk during
    subsequent intercourse)

Possibly safe/medium risk for transmission of infections
Oral sex with withdrawal before ejaculation, or with condom/
    dental dam
Vaginal intercourse with a condom
Anal intercourse with a condom
Urine externally on unbroken skin

Unsafe/high risk for STDs or HIV
Vaginal intercourse without a condom (risky for STDs, HIV and
    pregnancy)
Anal intercourse without a condom (risky for STDs and HIV)
Unprotected oral sex (risky for some STDs but lower or uncertain
    risk for HIV)
Rimming without latex protection
Drinking urine
Eating faeces
Sharing sex toys (theoretical risk of HIV)
Blood contact (theoretical risk of HIV)

What is safer sex? A more complex view

Public education has tended to focus on four issues that can affect the risk of infection with HIV:

• partner selection

• number of partners

• mode of sexual expression, i.e. types of sexual practice

• use of condoms.

However, while there is ample evidence that people are well informed about HIV transmission routes, it is less clear whether the public's understanding of the term 'safer sex' coincides with that intended by health educators. Research suggests that the public view of 'safer sex' is primarily to do with wearing condoms and reducing the number of partners. Few heterosexual people associate non-penetrative sex with 'safer sex', tending to think of such activities as preliminaries to penetration.

'Double-bind' messages, where there is a covert second message that contradicts the first, can lead to some confusion – especially the message often given to young people, 'Don't have sex, but if you do, use a condom'. There are also real problems with messages based on partner selection, since the criteria by which people are supposed to select 'safe' partners are usually unclear. Some people report that they consider themselves safe because they 'know' their partners. However, on closer examination, their interpretation of 'knowing' one's partner bears no relation to that intended by health promotion workers, i.e. knowing his or her sexual history.

Celibacy and monogamy can always be presented as options (although monogamy is *not* safe if the partner has been at high risk) but do not realistically address the sexual needs of many people. Safer sex messages based on 'only have unprotected sex with a partner you can trust' come up against problems with the public's understanding of 'trust'. For many people, *not* asking certain questions, for example about risk behaviour outside the relationship, may be more fundamental to a 'trusting' relationship than talking honestly and openly.

One approach is to take a positive stance of emphasizing risk reduction within a concept of 'healthy sexuality', rather than a stance that may be construed as 'sex-negative'. This may make it less likely that people will reject safer sex messages as being too restrictive, or that they will accept only those parts of the message that do not demand significant behavioural changes for them personally (e.g. 'It doesn't affect me, because I only have one partner... at a time').

Pros and cons of general practice as a setting for promoting sexual health

Advantages

- Reaches large numbers on a one-to-one level

- Relationship with patient already exists

- Opportunities to discuss sexual health arise during relevant consultations, for example for smears or contraception

- Setting is familiar to the patient and there is no stigma in being seen to attend

- Primary health care staff commonly deal with relationship problems

- Patient has permission to talk about any health concern and is not limited by particular specialist range

- Directly accessible when concerns arise

Disadvantages

- Limited time and increasing work-loads for staff

- Limited staff training on communication about sexuality and related issues

- Patients' and staffs' perceptions about the remit of primary care

- Fears of jeopardizing professional–patient relationship by raising sexual matters

- Concerns about confidentiality and record-keeping

- Embarrassment of staff in discussing sexuality, especially in consultations not directly related to sex

- Attitudes and values around sexuality and cultural issues

- Some groups, for example drug users and people with language difficulties, have difficulty accessing primary health care

- Some groups, for example fit young men, use primary health care infrequently

- Health promotion 'banding scheme' provides no financial incentive for sexual health work – although FHSAs can fund innovative work to address local priorities

The general practice setting

The key advantage of general practice as a setting for sexual health promotion is that it involves one-to-one consultations with very large numbers of people. Most people are registered with a GP, 60% consult each year and 80–90% consult at least once in every five years. However, some groups may need active targeting because they have difficulty in accessing primary care (e.g. injecting drug users) or rarely use this service (e.g. fit young men).

General practice is only one of many places where health promotion messages can be given. It is important for primary care staff to participate in wider campaigns, with posters, leaflets and readily available information, and also to capitalize on the particular features of the general practice setting by developing a personal style and approach to health promotion in individual consultations. These consultations can be important to individual clients, as there is potential for giving advice in a supportive and non-judgemental way and being open to answer questions that may arise.

Lack of time is a major problem for primary care professionals, and this can sometimes limit the extent of health promotion, in particular opportunistic health promotion. However, priorities can occasionally be redefined, and patients can be asked to make a return visit when an issue arises that requires attention and time. As with alcohol and smoking cessation, sexual health promotion can take time for some patients. For others, it can be a brief intervention designed to reinforce information received from other sources. The high status accorded to GPs and nurses by the public lends particular weight to the information and health promotion messages they give to patients.

It may be useful to point out that although staff in organizations starting to incorporate HIV into their work often express concern that HIV and sex will dominate work-loads and marginalize other activities, this rarely happens in reality. Skills such as 'closing interviews', which primary care professionals use to control their work-load in other circumstances, can equally well be applied to sexual health promotion.

Different staff roles and training

All members of the primary care team may be involved in sexual health promotion. For example, the way in which receptionists deal with requests for urgent appointments, especially from adolescents, is critical in creating a 'sexual health-friendly' environment. These patients may need emergency contraception or may be worried about symptoms of a possible STD. In some practices, receptionists distribute condoms, although this has raised concerns about patient privacy and confidentiality.

Different members of the primary health team may have different strengths in reaching various groups within the patient population. For example, nurses often carry out more planned health promotion and clinics that follow a set protocol, while doctors may be better placed to undertake opportunistic work with patients attending because of symptoms (whether related to sexual health or not). Some patients find it easier to discuss their concerns with a nurse, although for others it may be important to talk to a professional of their own sex, which can be a problem since most nurses are women. There is evidence that some primary care nurses feel under-utilized at present, and that with support and training, they would like to take a more proactive role in sexual health promotion. In addition to doctors and nurses, health visitors, midwives and counsellors can all be involved in sexual health promotion in ways which are appropriate to their distinct professional roles.

Staff team roles can be defined to prevent work being duplicated, and to identify which patients to target and when. It is useful to map existing staff roles, co-ordination and delineation between roles, and the ways in which staff roles complement each other, as a way of exploring how to develop and organize sexual health promotion. Practice guidelines, based on standards that have been agreed and documented, can be used for education and to ensure consistency between health professionals. Research shows that staff find guidelines help them to raise the subject of sexual health promotion opportunistically.[2] However, some professionals may find guidelines restrictive or a barrier to a patient-centred approach.

In general, primary health teams have a high level and broad range of skills. These skills may not be located specifically in sexual health but are often transferable. However, research consistently shows that staff lack confidence in discussing sex and sexual health with patients, suggesting a need for training and support.[3] Staff may benefit from training to develop knowledge, skills and attitudes relating to the following specific topics:

- knowledge about STDs, including HIV
- confidentiality, including how to deal with requests for information from insurers and mortgage lenders
- consent to HIV testing and treatment
- communication and counselling skills, including vocabulary and ways of raising the subject of sex and dealing with emotional issues
- sexual history-taking
- protocol and policy development
- team working
- working with men
- condoms: information on the range available and how to demonstrate their correct usage.

Opportunities for sexual health promotion

The waiting room

The ambience in the waiting room can set the tone for a whole practice. It is also a place to offer information in a way that may seem less threatening to people who are shy or embarrassed when talking about sex with a nurse or doctor. There is potential for:

- poster displays

- information updates on particular topics

- leaflets for people to help themselves

- positive images of young people, gay men, lesbians and drug users

- a practice newsletter with regular articles on sexual health

- it may be possible to provide condoms or, failing that, information on where to get free condoms

- anti-discrimination statement

- it may also be helpful to have a practice policy on confidentiality displayed with special reference to young people's right to confidentiality

---

There are many ways in which health promotion can happen, ranging from what takes place in individual consultations to the way the environment in which we practise affects our clients. Research shows that patients believe that it is appropriate to raise HIV prevention during many types of consultation, including wholly opportunistically, provided that presenting problems are dealt with first and that the patient is not in severe mental or physical distress.[4,5] Possibilities include new patient screening/registration, general check-ups, consultations relating to contraception, STDs and smears, pregnancy testing and travel clinics.

New patient registration examinations

This is an ideal time to include a brief sexual history, with the general medical history and recording of current problems and information for the health promotion banding scheme. New patients expect to be questioned about their health and life-style, so a context for sexual history-taking presents itself. A relationship has yet to be established between the health professional and the patient, so there is no fear of jeopardizing existing relationships. Raising sexual health at this time demonstrates a holistic approach and gives patients 'permission' to raise future worries, should these arise. Accurate sexual histories avoid assumptions about patients' sexual preferences, which could lead to inappropriate offers of contraceptive advice.

Contraception

Patients consulting for contraception expect to talk about sex and related concerns. Safer sex practices can be discussed, and condoms given if appropriate. One study found that although 90% of women would like to be able to discuss STDs (and HIV) when visiting their GP for family planning advice, only 10% had been able to do so.[6]

Well Woman/Well Man checks

Staff often identify these clinics as a time when sexual health promotion can be undertaken. As for new patient screening, sexual history-taking enables staff to avoid assumptions about patients' sexual preferences, demonstrates a holistic approach and gives patients 'permission' to raise future concerns.

Consultations concerning sexually transmitted diseases or where the patient raises the issue of his or her risk of HIV or STDs

This is a good time for health promotion work because both patient and health care professionals agree that the agenda is sexual behaviour. In this situation, it is relatively easy to address the subject but it is important not be be embarrassed, flustered or taken aback, and to listen carefully to the patient's concerns. It may be useful to:

- have a set of routine questions that allow you to assess the patient's risk (see section on sexual history-taking), and also prevent embarrassment and let the patient know that you are comfortable with the topic. Questions cover areas such as condom use, injecting drug use, numbers of partners, genitourinary symptoms, kinds of sex (i.e. anal or vaginal intercourse) and reasons for concern now

- have an open-minded approach, as discussed elsewhere in this book

- be able to provide information, for example on:
  - local genitourinary medicine (GUM) or sexual health clinics
  - likely investigations
  - likely treatments
  - voluntary sector provision, for example the Terrence Higgins Trust, Mainliners, Body Positive or Brook Advisory Centres
  - what is risky
  - what is safe

- be willing to write referral letters or make 'phone calls to ensure good hand-over to other health providers and make the patient's life easier

- if patients prefer not to go to the GUM clinic, have a strategy for investigation and treatment in the practice as a back-up (see Management of sexually transmitted diseases, Chapter 7). It may be worth discussing this with local GUM consultants, and it is best if it is uniform within the practice

- be willing to provide HIV testing and feel comfortable with test counselling for patients who feel they would rather have the test within the practice. Local health advisors may be willing to provide some training. It may be possible to arrange for the local laboratory to accept tests with only number codes, to emphasize the confidentiality of the test

- consider negotiating with your FHSA for free condoms (see Chapter 9).

Pregnancy and postnatal checks

Sexual problems as a result of delivery can easily be raised, and this is a time when patients expect contraception and related issues to be discussed.

Termination referral and counselling

This may be a difficult time to raise sensitive issues. However, with a good relationship and a sensitive approach, it may be possible.

Travel clinics

Patients are now aware of the high prevalence of STDs and HIV in many holiday destinations, so safer sex can be discussed in this context. The patient may have more time with the health care professional in this situation.

Sexual dysfunction

Details of any sexual problem raised by the patient need to be explored fully, together with a broader sexual history before treatment or referral.

Adolescent clinics

Adolescence is an ideal time to discuss sexual activity and safer sexual practices. Reassurances about confidentiality need to be given, and health professionals should actively seek ways to make the practice 'adolescent friendly', for example:

- giving information in the practice leaflet about confidentiality and services such as emergency contraception

- routinely asking teenage patients attending for other reasons about their emotional life and whether they have any concerns at school or at home, and emphasizing the willingness to help with worries, should they arise

- perhaps sending 'birthday card' appointments, inviting young people (e.g. at age 16) for a health check (enabling the recording of baseline data for the health promotion banding scheme) and the opportunity to discuss concerns. These need not relate only to sexual activity and relationships – acne, menstrual problems, weight and eating disorders, bullying, substance use, emotional distress and worries about education or employment prospects may also be important

- where appropriate, giving parents accompanying adolescent patients 'permission' to withdraw, so that the young person can talk with the professional in confidence

- publicizing local services for young people, so they have a choice of provider.

Chronic illness

The sexual well-being of a patient with a chronic illness is often over-looked. Sexual problems may result from the disease itself, med-ication or strain on a relationship owing to persistent ill health. These problems should be identified with a sexual history and dealt with as part of overall patient care.

Prescribing

Many drugs can affect sexual function; for example, beta blockers can cause impotence. These possible side-effects should be dis-cussed from the beginning. Other issues related to sexual health promotion may then present themselves.

Advice after myocardial infarction

Patients with diseases such as ischaemic heart disease often have concerns about physical exertion and sexual activity. Sensible advice, explanation and reassurance form part of sexual health promotion.

Opportunistic sexual health promotion for patients presenting
with unrelated conditions

This *is* possible, although health professionals may have difficulty in
raising the subject because of embarrassment or apprehensions about
how patients may react. Some tactics for raising the subject are sug-
gested in Chapter 3, 'Talking about sex'.

Other hints about how to manage this situation include:

- not getting carried away with the sexual health agenda and
  forgetting the patient's original problem

- developing a checklist for assessing sexual risk, which could
  come partly from information in the notes and partly from
  history-taking during the current consultation. This may cover
  age, sexual activity, use of contraception, drug use, foreign travel
  and other areas that seem relevant. It is important to become
  confident in using it and to trust the decision that is made based
  on it

- sometimes deciding not to raise the subject because of pressure
  of time or the complexity of the presenting problem. In this case,
  recording concern in the notes highlights the need to discuss
  sexual health on another occasion

- the importance of providing the opportunity for a follow-up consultation. Literature for patients to take away is also useful, as are
  free condoms if these are available.

How to target those at higher risk of HIV or sexually transmitted diseases

Great emphasis has been placed on health promotion and safer sex
information for the population at large. However, in the face of time
constraints, it is likely that we will all have to make choices about
whom to spend extra time with and whom to target for sexual health
promotion activities. If this is the case, we should focus on those with
the most to gain. This means those people who are running significant risks on a regular basis. In theory, this ought to be cost-
effective in the long term in improving sexual health and preventing
disease, although this remains to be proven. However, cost is not the

prime consideration, as disease prevention and good sexual health are a just goal in themselves.

What is high risk?

- Those at high risk of HIV are people having unprotected anal or vaginal sex with partners who may be HIV-positive. Since there is no easy way to know a partner's HIV status, it is best to assume that any partner of unknown status may be positive. Increasing one's number of partners increases the chance of one of them being positive. In addition, sharing drug injecting equipment is a high-risk activity.

- Because more gay men are HIV-positive, sex with a gay man is more risky as he is more likely to be already infected. However, there has been an increase in the heterosexual transmission of HIV, and this risk should not be ignored.

- The risk of STDs, especially chlamydia which can lead to in-fertility, is high for heterosexual sex.

Who should be targeted?

Chlamydia infection is most common in young women, particularly teenagers. *Young* gay men continue to have an increasing rate of HIV infection. In view of this, and the overall demography of STDs and HIV, the people we need to target are:

- young people who are already sexually active or about to become so

- injecting drug users

- gay men

- those with many sexual partners

- people who have sex abroad in areas where the prevalences of HIV and STDs are high.

To some extent, the ideas described under 'Opportunities for sexual health promotion', page 10, will be effective in reaching these groups, and do not represent major innovations over day-to-day practice.

Once these sorts of interventions become routine and comfortable, practices may want to expand their health promotion activity to seek out patients who are at risk of becoming infected with HIV or other STDs. To this end, new services need to be piloted, with specific client groups in mind. The exact areas a practice chooses to develop might depend on its interests and patient population. If the progress of innovations is carefully monitored, it will be possible to see which developments are successful and cost-effective, and to continue with these. A few suggestions for targeting groups of clients who do not otherwise visit GPs often are given below, but this is not by any means an exhaustive list, merely a beginning.

• A young person's clinic, possibly run as a drop-in. This might be staffed by a different doctor or nurse, maybe someone young, so that teenagers do not feel they are seeing the family doctor, which might make them embarrassed. This would ideally run out of school hours and encourage teenagers to see the health professional alone.

• An invitation in the practice leaflet for all patients offering a health MOT. This would cover all relevant areas of health promotion, including sexual health.

• A men's clinic, including safer sex and sexual health promotion, as well as more traditional areas, such as ischaemic heart disease and alcohol.

• A willingness to register injecting drug users, even if the GP decides against prescribing methadone. This needs to be coupled with a non-judgemental approach to these patients and possibly some flexibility around appointment times.

• Consider displaying the practice policy on confidentiality in the practice leaflet or on the wall in the surgery. This would cover young people (under 16s), and could encompass a non-discrimination statement.

Spreading the net outside general practice

In addition to innovations within practices, there is potential for working with other agencies providing services to people whose activities put them at risk of HIV and STDs. Collaboration can improve all the services and can create very useful links. Every area has a different patchwork of services, and co-operation takes time and effort. Liaison between services is further discussed in a later section of this book, but a couple of initial ideas are to:

• consider taking part in education in schools or even providing clinics, perhaps in conjunction with an organization such as the Brook Advisory Centres. There may also be a role for providing advice sessions in which no prescribing takes place

• collaborate with other services likely to meet these clients (e.g. needle exchanges, help lines and family planning clinics). This might involve accepting and making referrals, offering advice, taking part in training or even joint policy workshops, and generally fostering a good relationship. This is much easier when we understand how other organizations work and what their strengths and weaknesses are. It also helps when they understand general practice. To this end, the more co-operation and com-munication, the better.

2

Ethical considerations

What special ethical issues does sexual health promotion raise?

Primary health care professionals encounter ethical issues in all areas of their work, but sexual health promotion involves some special sensitivities.

- In health promotion, the professional may raise issues that the patient has not explicitly asked to be addressed. This implies a special obligation to recognize and address any anxieties that the health promotion message may raise, as well as dealing fully with investigation and treatment of the patient's presenting condition.

- Sex is a sensitive topic, and few people are used to frank discussion of their own sexual behaviour. Some behaviours may carry stigma or specific meanings for some patients.

- Because STDs are transmissible, they can affect people other than the patient him- or herself. Diagnosis of an STD may raise major issues about trust and fidelity within a relationship, as well as about the partner's health.

- Under-age sex is common, despite legal barriers, and health professionals need to be able to respond to this.

- HIV raises particularly difficult issues because:
  - it is a chronic and ultimately fatal condition surrounded by fear, misunderstanding and stigma
  - the absence of a cure means that, unlike with conventional STDs, infected persons can never put the diagnosis behind them and forget about it, for example when entering new sexual relationships or considering parenthood.

  –   people who (are thought to) have HIV infection face hazards
       of discrimination or harassment, for example in employment,
       housing and education, as well as specific problems with
       insurance.

For these reasons, primary care professionals need to be especially
aware of ethical concerns and patients' needs for confidentiality
when undertaking sexual health promotion.

Confidentiality and the practice team

Many people are wary of disclosing information about their sexual
behaviour or drug use. One of the main reasons that people concerned about these health issues do not ask their GPs for advice is the
perceived lack of confidentiality in the primary care setting. Patients'
understanding of 'confidentiality' may differ from that of the practice
team, and many people may not realize that information cannot be
provided to a third party outside the practice without their consent.
Thus, it is important to reassure patients about confidentiality and to
review what this means, for example who has access to information
and to medical records, or who may need to be told. If the doctors
within the practice regard it as essential to be able to share information among themselves, or with other members of the primary health
care team, then this should be explained to patients. If information
does need to be passed to a third party, for example a health professional outside the practice team, the reasons should be discussed
with the patient. Patients may need reassurance that the fax machine
is kept in a secure place accessible only to staff.

   Each patient's confidentiality needs may change over time and can
be reviewed according to his or her health or social status. For example, if an HIV-positive patient becomes symptomatic he or she
may agree to a social worker being informed in order to advise about
benefit entitlements.

Possible ways of reassuring patients about confidentiality

- A *statement* about confidentiality can be included in practice leaflets or shown in the waiting room. Although absolute
  confidentiality cannot be promised in all circumstances, this
  shows that the whole practice team has agreed on minimum
  standards for respecting confidentiality.

- Terms of confidentiality can be discussed with *new patients*
  when they register with the practice, so that they understand
  clearly who has access to their notes, the surgery's database and fax messages.

- The leaflet for young people *Private and confidential: talking
  to doctors* can be displayed in the waiting room; this can be
  obtained from Brook Advisory Centres or possibly from local
  health promotion departments.

- *Codes*, such as Soundex or patient numbers, can be used
  instead of names on *test request* forms.

- Another option may be to develop a written *practice policy
  on confidentiality*, agreed by and applying to everyone
  working in the practice. This could be made accessible to
  patients.

Record-keeping

It is helpful to discuss with patients what will be written in the notes
and how sensitive information, for example about risk behaviour or
past sexually transmitted infections, will be handled. Some patients
may prefer to have an informal discussion without details of risk behaviour being documented. However, it is essential to keep accurate
records of tests taken, results, follow-up and current clinical status in
order to provide effective treatment and continuity of care, especially
for ongoing conditions such as HIV infection. In most cases, being
open and honest about the importance of documenting information,

while emphasizing the practice team's sensitivity and commitment to confidentiality, will reassure patients that information will be kept safe, and that it is in their best interests to disclose it.

Where a patient has a transmissible infection, such as hepatitis B, it is important to explain that the reason for recording the specific diagnosis is to ensure appropriate treatment and care. If an infection hazard label is to be used, this may be placed on the inside cover of the notes where those staff who need to see it can do so, but it should be a general warning that does not name the specific infection concerned. Again, the reasons for this action should be explained to the patient.

Under the Access to Health Records Act 1990, people have the right to see their records, although there are exceptions for material that is liable to harm the patient's health or which might breach another person's confidentiality. Patients must not be given access to information that identifies another person, except another clinician. This means that health professionals should refuse to show patients any parts of their notes that mention a sexual partner's infection or risk status. Doctors who keep sensitive or speculative information separately from ordinary records should note that the Act applies to all medical records, including such special ones.

Young people

There is no legal or ethical barrier to asking young people under 16 about their sexual behaviour for health promotion purposes, but sensitivity is clearly needed as most have not had intercourse.[7] One approach may be to introduce the subject by saying something like, 'Because of the risks of AIDS and other infections we now ask all our patients about their sexual behaviour. This may be relevant to you now or in the future'.

Broadly speaking, people aged 16 or 17 have similar rights to confidentiality and to consent to investigation or treatment as an adult. People under 16 can seek medical advice and can consent to treatment, without their parents' knowledge, provided the health professional judges that they are able to understand the choices open to them, including the nature, purpose and risks of treatment. However, a doctor consulted about contraception by a person under 16 has a duty to encourage the patient to inform his or her parents about the consultation and to explore the reasons if the patient is unwilling to do so. *If a patient aged under 16 refuses parental involvement, confidentiality should be maintained,* even if treatment has been refused on the grounds that the patient is too immature to consent to it. This right to confidentiality should be emphasized to young patients, for example in practice literature, although there can be rare exceptions in cases of sexual abuse or exploitation.

Confidentiality and insurance

GPs are often asked to provide reports to a patient's insurance company or employer. Such reports cannot be given without the patient's consent, and the patient has a right to see them under the Access to Medical Reports Act 1988.

The golden rule is that, in writing a report, the GP should stick to factual, clinical information and avoid speculation or hearsay. It is best to refuse to answer questions about patients' life-styles or risks of acquiring HIV.[a]

There has been considerable confusion over the insurance implications of being tested for HIV. Fortunately, the Association of British Insurers has now advised companies *not* to ask applicants for life insurance whether they have ever been counselled or tested about HIV or STDs. This change may substantially increase people's willingness to discuss sexual behaviour and concerns about HIV with members of the primary care team. People who have tested positive for HIV or STDs may still have to disclose this fact, and those with HIV infection will ordinarily be refused insurance. Where a GP is asked to report on whether a person is HIV-positive or has had an STD, the doctor should do so accurately on the basis of information recorded in the notes. Applicants for large amounts of insurance will continue to be required to be tested and/or to answer life-style questions.

---

[a] Stickers to put on the report form saying 'BMA guidance states: It is essential that a doctor does not speculate about the patient's lifestyle or "risk" of HIV infection. Such questions can only be answered by the patient and the insurance company should be directed to seek the information from the patient him/herself', can be obtained from Sheffield Centre for HIV and Sexual Health, 22 Collegiate Crescent, Sheffield S10 2BA.

Consent to testing for STDs and HIV infection

Aims of HIV test counselling

• To ensure the person understands the nature of the test and its implications so that he or she can make an informed decision on whether or not to consent to testing (pre-test).

• To support the person in preparing for and coping with the emotional impact of the test result and its health and social implications (pre- and post-test).

• To enable the person to assess his or her risk of exposure to HIV and to adopt risk-reduction strategies that suit his or her individual circumstances and life-style (pre- and post-test).

Explicit informed consent is necessary before testing for STDs or HIV, in view of the serious implications of some infections. For example, a positive test result for HIV antibodies or chronic hepatitis B infection can severely affect a patient's psychological well-being, and may result in discrimination and affect personal relationships, as well as financial circumstances. These issues can be covered alongside the direct health implications of the infection during pre-test discussion.

Moreover, providing patients with information about tests can be an opportunity to reinforce advice about risk reduction and their responsibility for their own health, as well as to enable them to understand which infections can be transmitted to others and how to prevent this.

It is essential that the health professional who undertakes the pre-test discussion is familiar with the meaning of the test, its accuracy and the possible risks and benefits of being tested. For HIV antibody testing, it can be helpful to ask the patient to sign in the medical notes to indicate that he or she has consented to the test after receiving pre-test counselling or discussion and having the implications explained.

Some practices use Soundex codes (a way of encoding a person's initial and surname) or patient numbers instead of names on test request forms to ensure confidentiality. The PHLS Communicable Disease Surveillance Centre can provide written information on how to use Soundex, or a coding program that will run on most computers.

Ideally, health workers should treat all blood samples as potentially infectious, but many laboratories require samples from patients deemed to be at high risk of infection to be specially labelled. It is important to explain to patients why such (non-disease specific) labels are needed.

Partners of patients with HIV or STDs who may be at risk from infection

For many infections, the patient's sexual partner(s) should be contacted to attend for information, tests and possible treatment. Contact tracing, or partner notification, is generally regarded as essential for gonorrhoea, syphilis and chancroid, but should also be carried out for chlamydia and other infections. The General Medical Council advises that doctors must discuss with a patient who is found to be HIV positive the question of informing sexual partners. It is often advisable to raise this issue in pre-test discussion, so that the patient is prepared in advance.

If the importance is explained to them, most patients will agree to inform partners who may be at risk of infection, especially current partners. However, they may require support and encouragement from the GP when doing so, especially where this could affect the stability of the relationship. Engaging in role play to allow the patient to 'rehearse' how he or she will inform the partner and offering to be at hand and available for immediate consultation after the partner has been informed are ways of helping.

However, if patients do not want to inform their contacts themselves, they may ask a health professional to do so, or the GP may offer. GPs may want to consider in advance how they will deal with such a situation, bearing in mind that they have an obligation to help those patients who are willing for their partners to be informed. For example, the GP could refer the patient to the GUM clinic, whose health advisers can assist in partner notification. Patients should be reassured that partners will not be told their identity and, other than for HIV, will not be told the specific diagnosis, but merely that they may have been exposed to a sexually transmitted disease. Where the partner is a patient of the GP, however, it may be more appropriate for the GP to contact him or her directly to make an appointment at the surgery.

Situations occasionally arise in which patients refuse to inform current sexual or drug injecting partners. The General Medical Council has said that a doctor may consider informing a partner without the patient's explicit consent, if he or she believes that there is 'a serious and identifiable risk to a specific individual who, if not informed, would be exposed' to HIV infection. If the doctor decides that such a breach of confidentiality would be justified, he or she should inform the patient in advance before notifying the partner(s), and should seek to support the patient throughout.

Referring to other specialists

Many patients with sexual health problems can be adequately treated in primary care, but it may sometimes be more appropriate to refer to a GUM department, family planning clinic, young people's advisory clinic or specialist in psychosexual medicine. For example, some people at a higher risk of acquiring infections may require extensive counselling about unsafe sexual or drug use behaviour. Referral for contact tracing may also be appropriate, as discussed above, as clinics can provide greater anonymity and employ health advisers who can counsel patients about sexually transmitted infections.

Some GPs consider referral to a GUM clinic appropriate for patients who request HIV testing, since clinic staff may have more experience of pre- and post-test counselling. In such cases, it is wise for the GP to explain to the patient why he or she is being referred and to stress that the GP is interested in knowing the test results and in taking part in follow-up and possible shared care with the clinic. Otherwise, patients may misconstrue a referral as a form of rejection and an indication that the GP is unwilling to care for people with HIV.

Referral is important in the management of patients with some infections, such as active hepatitis B and HIV, for which specialist assessment is needed. However, since HIV is a chronic condition, with intermittent acute episodes, subsequent follow-up can be provided by the GP in liaison with the specialist unit.

When making any referral, the GP can specifically request the clinic to send summaries of clinic visits so that the primary care team is kept informed (providing the patient consents) about anything which may affect the patient's care.

Attitudes to sex and sexuality

One of the barriers to sexual health promotion is the hypocritical nature of British society. The media exploits sexuality and sex through film, television, literature and music, yet sex is viewed as a private and hidden affair, if not a little embarrassing, especially to talk about on a personal level. Barriers to talking about sexual health include attitudes, myths, prejudices and taboos such as:

• the notion that sex is only for procreation, which negates the role of sex as a source of pleasure and an expression of intimacy, love and emotional closeness

• assumptions about male and female sex roles and prescriptive heterosexuality, which can create conflicts for individuals between their internal feelings and the way in which they are expected to behave in society

• denial of sexuality in childhood – the way in which children's sexual behaviour is viewed can promote openness about sexuality or create guilt and shame from an early age.

Health professionals encounter the full range of human diversity in their work, and should be able to meet the needs of all patients without discrimination. Fundamental to this is the ability to recognize sexual diversity and to avoid stereotyping patients, for example not to assume that everyone is heterosexual unless they fit a gay or lesbian stereotype. Professionals are often instructed to be 'non-judgemental' at all times, but this is arguably an unattainable ideal. It is more realistic to accept that we all have prejudices and that we need to explore them before attempting to offer patients 'non-judgemental' care. Thus, health professionals may find it easier to accept others in all their sexual diversity if they can first acknowledge their own sexuality and understand how it has been shaped by biological, psychological and social factors. The processes of professional development whereby health workers can explore their own attitudes are covered in more depth later in this book, in Chapter 11, on Professional development.

3

Talking about sex

Raising the issue

Raising the issue of sexual health, especially opportunistically, can be difficult in primary care. Although a recent survey found that 98% of general practices offered a family planning and GUM referral service with advice on safer sex, actual uptake was low.[8] Many GPs were prepared to give advice about safer sex, but only did so when requested by the patient and not as a routine part of contraceptive consultations.

In family planning and GUM clinics, the setting provides legitimization to talk about sexual behaviour, but this is not the case in general practice, unless the patient presents with a clearly sex-related concern. It may be reassuring to know that some professionals with considerable experience in specialist sexual health services (e.g. GUM) still find it difficult to initiate discussion of sex in a general practice setting.

Staff vary in the ease and comfort with which they can discuss sexual activities. In one study, 26% of GPs said they felt uncomfortable when talking to patients about explicit sexual matters.[1] Similarly, 10% of community nurses said they felt uneasy when discussing sexual matters, rising to 20% for discussing HIV.[3] It has been shown that staff with more experience of patients with HIV infection are more confident at giving sexual health education.[9] Training in communication skills and knowledge of safer sex practices can also enable staff to feel more confident. The English National Board for Nursing, Midwifery and Health Visiting has developed a specific training package on sexual health for nurses, which offers many useful insights for other professional groups as well.

Staff may fear that patients will regard sexual health as outside their remit, or feel that it is intrusive to be asked about sexual activities. Such fears are generally misplaced: research shows that patients regard it as appropriate for GPs and practice nurses to take sexual histories.

Familiarity between staff and patients may help discussion around sensitive issues. However, some patients prefer the anonymity of GUM or other outside clinics. Staff can reassure patients about the confidentiality that exists in general practice, but should also accept that some patients will choose to go elsewhere.

Tactics that may make it easier to raise the subject of sexual health with patients include the following.

• Practice protocols or guidelines can be developed that target specific consultations for sexual health promotion to give staff a clear framework.

• A 'hook' or 'excuse' can be used, for example, 'Because World AIDS Day(1 December)/Valentine's Day/the holiday season/Christmas is coming up, we're having a special focus this week on sexual health. Do you have any concerns you would like to raise about your relationships and sex life, or about AIDS?'

• Advertising the sexual health services provided at the practice may encourage patients to raise concerns. This can include a display of posters and leaflets in the waiting area and consultation rooms, or outlining sexual health services in the practice leaflet. Publicity also provides staff with a useful prompt for initiating discussion ('What do you think about the poster?').

• Having condoms available will enable the professional to feel that he or she has something to offer to patients (see Chapter 9, on Providing condoms).

• Routine sexual history-taking can also be used as a hook: 'Because of concerns about HIV/AIDS, we now ask all our patients about their sexual behaviour and life-style…'. It is particularly valuable to incorporate this approach into consultations that follow a set pattern or protocol, for example new patient screening, Well Woman/Well Man/adolescent clinics (see Opportunities for sexual health promotion, Chapter 1).

Taking sexual histories

> If people who practise high-risk behaviour are to be identified, sexual histories need to be incorporated into general medical history-taking. Certain factors, for example open-ended quesions, summarizing frequently, clarification and negotiation, can improve the quality of information gathered. This demonstrates the importance of training primary health care professionals to take sexual histories. However, it is equally important to recognize that primary health care professionals already routinely use many of the necessary skills in other areas of their work.

There are clear benefits to both patient and professional in taking a sexual history. This is an important element in building a complete picture of a patient and planning appropriate management. A holistic approach to sexual history-taking is advocated, following on from the medical and social history. There are several key benefits to taking a sexual history.

- It gives patients permission to raise concerns and questions regarding their sexual health, at that time or in the future.

- It enables safer sex information and sexual health advice to be tailored to the individual patient's behaviour and life-style.

- It can identify patients who may be at increased risk of STDs, including HIV, so that resources can be targeted towards them. For example, if it is decided to target according to the patient's sexual preference or number of partners, this information cannot be obtained without taking a sexual history.

- It may increase the uptake and quality of STD screening, diagnosis and treatment in general practice or through referral to other services.

- It can improve the quality of contraceptive services by tailoring information on the advantages and disadvantages of different methods to the individual patients, to support them in choosing an appropriate method.

Obviously, the structure and content of a sexual history may vary depending on the circumstances of the consultation. However, there are some general pointers.

- The key to effective sexual history-taking is communication, which involves actively listening to patients and allowing time for them to say why they have attended and what they want. An awareness of body language is important, as it may both give messages to the patient and reveal information about the patient, through changes of speech pattern, tone of voice, downcast eyes, shifts in posture, etc. Sometimes, there may be a large discrepancy between what is said and what is communicated non-verbally, the non-verbal portion often being more accurate.

- It may be wrong to assume that if a patient exhibits discomfort, this means that he or she does not want the discussion to continue. However, professionals need to be aware of patients' feelings and to allow them to 'pass' on specific questions or to cease the discussion altogether.

- Interview techniques, such as reflecting back – 'So the issue is ...' or 'You mentioned that ...' – work well in obtaining more information. Summarizing what has been said so far gives the patient an opportunity to elaborate on a topic.

- Open questions are important to enable patients to express their concerns. Examples might be simply, 'Can you tell me a bit more about why you have come to see me?' or 'How are your relationships and sex life at the moment?'

- Closed questions can be used to elicit specific information but may result in inaccurate responses, especially if they relate to sensitive issues, such as anal sex or sexual preference. It is good practice to structure the history by starting with easier questions, to build trust before moving on to more private and difficult ones.

- Generalized statements, for example 'Many people are concerned about ...' or 'Many people experience...' can help patients to discuss sensitive issues more comfortably.

- Statistical questions, such as 'How many times a week do you have sexual intercourse?', may make patients want to give answers that show they are 'normal' or 'average', rather than providing accurate information.

- It is imperative not to make premature judgements about the person's sexual preference or behaviour. If questions are so phrased that they carry an assumption of heterosexuality, a patient may find it difficult to indicate that he or she is gay, lesbian or bisexual. It is wise to ask about 'partners' instead of husbands, wives, girlfriends or boyfriends.

- If the patient does not make his or her sexual preference clear, then the question, 'When did you last have sex and with whom?' is open-ended but may clarify the situation. If necessary it can be followed up with, 'And, can I check, is [your partner] a man or a woman?' Bisexuality, which is often hidden, also needs to be considered.

- Occasionally, heterosexual patients may be upset by an approach that raises the possibility of their being homosexual. The professional should be sensitive to such feelings, but not to the extent of failing to obtain relevant information, and should avoid encouraging or colluding with prejudices held by the patient. Reassurance can be given along the lines of, 'I need to ask these questions in order to help you; it's a routine question we ask our patients. We offer equal care and consideration to everyone, whether homosexual or heterosexual'.

- Vocabulary needs to be unambiguous. It helps if professionals are familiar with colloquial as well as medical terminology, but this does not mean that colloquial language, especially the cruder terms, should necessarily be used with patients. Some professionals recommend the use of medical vocabulary, whereas others suggest that vocabulary should be adapted to reflect that of the patient. Generally, as long as terms are defined, explained and shared, the best approach is the one the professional is most comfortable with.

- When talking to patients with learning difficulties, it is important to clarify the meaning of both words the patient uses and those used by the professional, otherwise patients may sometimes incorrectly assume the meaning of words, rather than expose their lack of understanding by asking for clarification. People with learning disabilities may also communicate through their actions, and it can take time to interpret the meaning of this and to create trust between the client and the professional.

It is also worth remembering that sexual feelings continue into extreme *old age* for many people. Professionals need to be aware of elderly patients' sexual health concerns in order to offer holistic care.

• Because of societal attitudes, older people may feel guilt about having sexual thoughts and feelings so it is important to give them 'permission' to raise concerns and to handle the issue sensitively.

• It should not be assumed that because a person is elderly, he or she must be heterosexual.

Practical suggestions for discussing sex

General screening history (e.g. new patients, Well Woman/ Well Man clinic)

How are your relationships and sex life?
And are you currently sexually active?
Do you have any worries or difficulties about having sex?
And are you in a relationship at the moment? (Not: And are you married/do you have a girlfriend/boyfriend? If unclear, follow up by checking whether partner is a man or a woman)
And do you have sex with anyone apart from your partner... and is that with men or women or both?
Do you have a need for contraception? (If appropriate, to be followed up by: What contraception do you use?)
Would you like any advice about safer sex and preventing AIDS and other diseases?

Asking about specific behaviours

When you have sex, what exactly do you do? ...And do you do anything else, as well as that?
Do you have vaginal intercourse? ...With or without a condom?
Do you have anal intercourse? ...With or without a condom?
Do you do [such and such]? ...Have you done so in the past? (Not: Do you ever...? or Have you ever...? – the word 'ever' conveys a suggestion that the behaviour is unusual and invites the answer 'No')

Use simple language and check for understanding, for example
Do you put your penis in his or her mouth? (Not: Do you
practise fellatio?)

Awareness raising

What do you know about how HIV is transmitted? …How can you
protect yourself? (Asking questions to assess the patient's
existing knowledge and opinions helps the professional to
pitch advice at an appropriate level and leads people to
identify solutions that are appropriate for them)
Would you like to talk about safer sex? or What do you know
about safer sex? (Not: Do you practise safer sex? – This
assumes a shared understanding of what safer sex is, which
may be lacking)
In what ways have you changed your behaviour because of HIV
and AIDS? (This is a deliberately leading question, intended
to stimulate people to think about whether or not they are at
risk)

One reason that GPs and practice nurses may be reluctant to take
sexual histories is for fear of opening a 'Pandora's box' of sexual
health need. At times, the most appropriate action may be to enable
patients to express their concerns, or have their symptoms diagnosed,
and then to offer another appointment at a later date or a referral to
an appropriate agency. However, successful referral depends on reducing the stigma associated with specialist sexual health services,
and enabling patients to recognize the benefits of using them. It is
important for patients to understand that there are many STDs (rather
than just HIV), which can be asymptomatic through a great deal of
their natural history but which can lead to significant morbidity or
even mortality. Examples include chlamydial pelvic inflammatory
disease causing ectopic pregnancy via tubal damage, hepatitis B
infection leading to hepatoma, subclinical wart virus infections leading to cervical intraepithelial neoplasia, and treponemal infection
leading to late clinical manifestations of syphilis. Ways in which general practice can help to defuse stigma associated with specialist
sexual health clinics include:

• providing brief information for patients about what happens at
the GUM clinic

- ensuring that all staff, including receptionists, have up-to-date information about local services, such as psychosexual counselling, GUM, termination and associated counselling, family planning clinics and specialist services for young people.

Components for history-taking in patients with symptoms of possible STD

Details of symptom(s)

- Duration

- Character

- Anatomical location

- Periodicity

- Relationship to sexual intercourse

- Whether similar symptoms have been experienced previously

The most common symptoms are urethral discharge and/or dysuria in men, and altered vaginal discharge in women. A complaint of 'vaginal discharge' does not always indicate pathology – physiological discharges can occur, for example at times of hormonal change.

Risk assessment

- Any previous STDs: whether diagnosis was confirmed, how and where they were treated, whether other tests, for example serology, were also performed

- Sexual history: preference, number of current and former partners, age of first sexual activity

- Sexual practices, orifices used – to identify sites for examination and culture

- Whether or not barrier contraception, spermicide or other protection used

---

- Whether partner(s) born or lived in specific endemic areas – for example for HIV, hepatitis B, penicillin-resistant gonococci

- Date of last exposure (NB: For infections diagnosed by serology, there is a need to judge whether the person could still be in the window period before seroconversion)

For HIV, risk assessment also includes whether the person has:

- Previously had an HIV test, and when

- Had a partner thought to be a current or former injecting drug user

- Injected drugs – whether needles were shared, and when drugs were last used

- Had a blood transfusion

- Donated blood (NB: This carries no risk of HIV. However, recipients need to be traced if a former donor of blood, semen, tissues or organs tests positive)

General

- Brief general medical history

- In women, gynaecological, contraceptive and obstetric history, date of last menstrual period and whether this was normal, periodicity of menstrual cycle and date of last cervical smear

Management

- At points during the history, re-emphasize confidentiality and feed back to the patient on the significance of information gained so far

- Summarize the assessment of likely risk at the end

- Discuss safer sex in context, reflecting the reality of the patient's life

- Obtain fully informed consent for tests and physical examination

- Inform the patient when and how to obtain results – to be given in person by a named individual

- De-brief, sum up and arrange any treatment, referrals or follow-up appointments

Transcultural working

Culture and religion influence people's sexuality in different ways. It may sometimes be useful to know a patient's religion when discussing his or her sexual or reproductive history. For example, if a patient attending for post-abortion counselling is a Roman Catholic, her religion may raise specific issues for her. However, there is a fine line between cultural sensitivity and cultural stereotype, and it is important that the health professional's knowledge and assumptions about a patient's culture or religion do not dictate the content or nature of the consultation. A person's beliefs may or may not match his or her actual behaviour.

Many primary care professionals have concerns about working with patients whose culture and religion differ from their own, and not only in the context of sexual health. If in doubt, the best approach is to ask the patient, for example by saying 'Is it OK to talk about sex?' This gives patients an opportunity to indicate whether or not they feel it appropriate to discuss such matters. Even if a patient does not wish to discuss his or her personal sexuality, it may sometimes be possible to give practical advice in general terms, for example information about safer sex or STDs and HIV transmission. Moreover, simply asking patients whether they wish to discuss sexual matters or are permitted to do so by their faith is a useful first step in raising awareness and signalling the professional's willingness to address any concerns they might have in future.

Developing practice guidelines on sexual history-taking

The following questions are intended to aid practice teams in developing their own guidelines on when and how to take sexual
histories, or to clarify their existing practice. They can be considered in the context of general work, or specific consultations and clinics, for example Well Woman/Well Man,
contraception or new patient screening.

What is your current sexual history-taking practice?
What strengths and weaknesses are there in your practice?
In what ways could your sexual history-taking be improved
further?

Which are the times when you would/would not take a sexual
history?
And are there particular patients from whom you would/would
not take a sexual history?
What blocks might exist to your sexual history-taking?
What would help to overcome these?

How confidential is the service, and what will you tell the patient
about this?

When will you introduce the subject of sexual history?
From whom will you take a sexual history?
What questions will you ask?
Why will you ask those questions?
How will you follow through on the information you receive?
To which referral agencies could you refer patients?
What information might you want to give the patient?
How will you record the information you receive?

Do you require any further information?
Where could you get this information from?

Do you require any further skills development?
Where could you get assistance to develop your skills?

Some issues relating to gay and bisexual men

The HIV/AIDS epidemic has focused attention on the sexual health needs of gay and bisexual men, since around 60% of reported cases of HIV infection in the UK up to the end of 1994 have been attributed to sexual contact between men, yet many health professionals have little specific training in this area. In one study, only 12% of general practice trainees and 21% of trainers found it easy to discuss sex with male homosexual patients; this contrasts with 70% of trainees who felt able to undertake the arguably more difficult task of counselling patients wanting HIV testing.[10] Another study[11] found that although over 90% of a sample of homosexual men were registered with GPs and over 80% had consulted in the previous year, only 56% of those who were registered said that their doctor knew about their sexual preference. Most of these had volunteered the information rather than being asked. However, 84% of the sample regarded GPs as an appropriate source of safer sex advice for gay men. (In addition, 44% of the men who knew themselves to be HIV positive had not informed their GP of this, and, of these, more than one-third had consulted their GP in the past year.) This suggests that it may be necessary to reassure gay men that they will get a sympathetic and confidential reception in general practice, but that once this is done, valuable health advice can be given. Steps that may help include:

• advertising the practice's policy on confidentiality and non-discrimination in leaflets, posters, etc. and stressing this when talking with patients

• taking sexual histories, avoiding language that assumes hetero-sexuality and, where appropriate, asking patients whether they are homosexual or heterosexual, in a simple and neutral manner

• if a patient refers to an aspect of homosexual practice or life-style that is unfamiliar to you, there is no harm in simply asking him or her to explain it

• being sensitive to the fact that patients may already know a great deal about HIV, may have lost friends through AIDS, or may know themselves to be HIV positive.

At times, the fact that gay men have been disproportionately affected by HIV/AIDS has been used as an excuse for blame and prejudice, instead of an occasion to examine the health *needs* of gay men and how best these can be met. Yet a 1992 survey[12] found a striking absence of HIV prevention work specifically for gay men, suggesting that primary care teams should not assume that these needs are being adequately met by other services. Of course, as for anyone else, gay men's sexual health concerns may not be confined to HIV, but may include issues such as the impact of physical illness on sexual functioning, psychosexual and relationship difficulties, and other STDs. In addition, mental health problems may result from the stress of coming to terms with one's sexual identity in a society that is often openly hostile towards homosexuality. This may be particularly true for adolescents growing up gay or bisexual.[13]

The reasons for gay and bisexual men being disproportionately affected by HIV/AIDS in the UK are not entirely clear and may relate to patterns of sexual mixing and partner change, as well as to the ease of transmission of HIV through anal compared with vaginal intercourse. (It is important to note here that some heterosexuals practise anal intercourse, and some homosexual men do not.) Whatever the underlying reasons, gay men who practise unsafe sex are at higher risk of acquiring HIV infection than are heterosexuals with comparable patterns of sexual behaviour, simply because there is a higher prevalence of infection among gay men and thus a greater probability of selecting a partner who is already infected. This is illustrated in Table 3.1, which shows the prevalences of HIV infection found by anonymized screening of different groups of patients attending GUM clinics in 1993. However, among both homosexuals and heterosexuals, clinic attenders may not be representative of the population as a whole.

A basic understanding of homosexual identity, life-styles and practice can aid primary care professionals in offering appropriate and sensitive services. A major longitudinal survey of gay and bisexual men in England and Wales, known as Project Sigma,[15,16] points to the following key conclusions.

• Most gay men recognize that they are gay early in adolescence, and before they first have sex with another boy or man. Among survey participants, the mean age at first homosexual experience was 15.7 years, and the mean age at first anal intercourse was 20.9 years. There was no evidence that boys 'became' homosexual as a result of 'recruitment' by older men – 60% had their first homosexual experience with a partner within two years of their own age. Most

Table 3.1: Prevalence of HIV infection in different groups of GUM clinic attenders in 1993, excluding those known to inject drugs[14]

	London and South East		Rest of England and Wales	
	Mean % prevalence	Range of % prevalence between clinics	Mean % prevalence	Range of % prevalence between clinics
Homosexual/ bisexual men	15.79	3.61–21.36	4.31	0.73–8.24
Heterosexual men	0.97	0.08–1.86	0.11	0–0.30
Heterosexual women	0.57	0.28–1.16	0.09	0–0.49

hoped for their first such experience, and many actively sought it.

• Over 90% of the men chose to describe themselves as 'gay', including some who had sex with women as well as with men. 22% were 'out' (open about their sexual identity) with all their family, friends and work-mates, while 32% were 'out' with fewer than half of these. However, the sampling method may have over-represented men who identified more strongly as gay, missing those who regard themselves as heterosexual but also have sex with men.

• At any time, about 60% of men in the study had a regular sexual partner, although more than half of these also had sex with other (regular or casual) partners. One man in 20 had a regular female partner. The median length a relationship had lasted was 21 months, with a range of up to 38 years.

• Over the four waves of the longitudinal study (1987–91), there were substantial changes in individual behaviour, both towards safer and towards more risky behaviour:

   – with regular partners: 60% of men had no unprotected anal intercourse in any wave; 10% had unprotected anal intercourse throughout; 15% increased their risk, either by starting to have anal intercourse or by starting to do so without

condoms; 15% decreased their risk, either by stopping having anal intercourse or by starting to use condoms

- with casual partners: 76% had no unprotected intercourse in
any wave; 1% had unprotected intercourse throughout; 12%
increased their risk; 11% decreased their risk.

- The main determinant of whether an individual man's sexual
behaviour changed between different waves of the study was
whether or not his relationship(s) changed. Changes in risk
behaviour within an existing relationship were relatively rare.

- The most commonly reported sexual acts were masturbation of
self or partner, fellatio and kissing. Although over 90% of the
men had had anal intercourse at some time in their lives, 29%
had not done so in the year up to interview.

- The idea of 'active' and 'passive' homosexuals is largely a myth.
Most men who practise anal intercourse do so in both insertive
and receptive roles.

- Of the small number of men who acquired HIV infection during
the course of the study, most did so through unprotected anal
intercourse *with a regular partner*. This reflects the fact that unprotected intercourse was much more common with regular than
with casual partners. HIV prevention (whether effective or not) is
not the only reason why anal intercourse (either with or without
a condom) is often confined to regular partnerships; anal intercourse may have special emotional significance for many men.

- Very few men who enjoy anal intercourse have ceased to practise
it because of HIV. This accords with the special emotional status
of anal sex. It suggests that it is unrealistic to expect men who
want anal intercourse to give up such a powerful experience. It
may mean that health advice should focus on using condoms
and on choosing carefully with whom to have anal sex, rather
than on avoiding anal intercourse. Since a regular relationship is
not necessarily safe, HIV testing of both partners may be
considered as a way to assess the risk attached to anal sex for a
given couple.

The language of sex

Anilingus: Rimming, reaming. Oral–anal contact, licking, kissing or sucking the anus

Anal intercourse: Butt fucking, arse fucking, back or rear entry, buggering. Sexual intercourse where a person puts a penis or a sex toy inside the anus of a woman or a man

Anus: Arsehole, bumhole

Bondage: When people tie or chain one another up for sexual pleasure

Clitoris: Love button, clit. A small sensitive organ at the top of where the labia minora of the vagina meet. It plays a crucial role in the female orgasm

Cunnilingus: Licking, going down on, oral sex. Using the mouth and tongue to stimulate the labia and clitoris

Faeces: Shit, scat, brown. Sexual activities that involve faeces

Fellatio: Cock sucking, blow job, French, giving head, go down on, oral sex. Using the mouth and tongue to stimulate a man's penis

Fisting: Fist fucking, hand balling. Inserting the hand into another person's vagina or rectum

Massage: Caressing and stroking the body for sensual or sexual enjoyment or relaxation. Aromatherapy oils may be used

Mutual masturbation: Hand job. Using hands to stimulate each others' genitals at the same time or in turn

Oral sex: Using the mouth and tongue to stimulate another person's genitals

Penis: Dick, prick, knob, willy, plonker, cock, shaft, John Thomas, old boy, Ram Rod

Sado-masochism: S/M. Obtaining erotic stimulation through giving or receiving physical or psychological pain and/or humiliation

'Sixty nine': A term for mutual oral sex

Vagina: Cunt, fanny, mary, minnie, pussy, minge, muff

Vaginal intercourse: Fucking, bonking, shagging, penetration, screwing, 'having sex', 'making love'. Sexual intercourse in which a person puts a penis or sex toy into a woman's vagina

Watersports: Golden showers, pissing, yellow. Sexual activities that involve urine

Sex toys: Vibrators, fruit and vegetables, strap-on dildo. 'Toys' that are used either for personal sexual pleasure or with another person

Partner management

'Partner management' can cover a spectrum of activities, from formal contact tracing for patients with definite STDs through to more general support to enable patients who wish to do so to discuss risks and behaviour change with their partners. Patients should be encouraged to make an informed choice about whether to divulge personal sexual health details to their partners. Practitioners should not tell patients what to do as regards talking to their partners but they can make helpful suggestions, such as how to approach a sensitive subject such as safer sex with a partner. It is often difficult for patients to make changes in behaviour, and they may not want to offend a partner and risk losing him or her. However, patients have to take responsibility for any compromises they make regarding their sexual health.

Before beginning to counsel patients about talking to their partners, the practitioner must first establish the nature of the relationship(s) involved, if the patient feels comfortable disclosing this. Assumptions about relationships should be avoided – married people are not all monogamous, and people in heterosexual relationships can have same-sex relationships that are known or unknown to their opposite-sex partners.

When counselling patients about talking to their partners, the professional may begin by explaining that there are several aspects of sexual communication, for example making sexual statements, making requests and dealing with conflict and negotiation.

The professional can help the patient to talk to his or her partners by giving practical advice, for example:

- the need to be prepared for the partner to react in a variety of possible ways, from willingness to objection, resistance and denial. Patients should also consider whether it is safe to raise the issue with a partner, or whether there may be an aggressive or violent reaction

- choosing a good time to raise the subject, when both partners will be reasonably calm and free of interruptions

- creating an atmosphere in which both partners can talk in a relaxed, unhurried fashion

- possible opening lines such as 'I'd like to talk to you about safer sex' or 'I was discussing sexual health with the doctor/nurse today', and developing the conversation from there

- finding ways of negotiating solutions to sexual health problems that are acceptable, realistic and desirable for both partners by:

    - avoiding apportioning blame between themselves and their partners

    - joining together with their partner, for example saying, 'What are we going to do about this?' rather than, 'What are you going to do?'

    - taking a positive approach, for example 'I'd like it if you would...', rather than 'You never...'

    - making decisions about behaviour change by mutual consent, so that both partners share responsibility.

Some patients may ask to be seen together with their partner to discuss sexual health with the professional, as such a formal setting can provide a safety net for the couple. A practitioner who agrees to such a consultation should attempt to initiate dialogue between the partners, rather than doing all the talking him or herself. It takes particular skills to facilitate couple counselling in this way, and GPs or practice nurses should only take on this role if they feel confident in doing so.

4

Psychosexual problems

The reassuring thing to remember is that although this may not be an area of special interest or further training for most GPs, there is nothing 'special' about the communication skills required to deal with psychosexual problems. The practitioner should be reassured that he or she is unlikely to add to the patient's problems by staying within the patient's level of disclosure on general questioning.

- Finding out the patient's expectations can be very helpful. We, as health professionals, often feel that patients expect more than we can deliver. In this area, in particular, it can be reassuring to us to know what is expected. It is often a lot less than we imagine. If patients have unrealistic expectations – commonly, that there is a blood test that will reveal all, or a tablet that will cure all – an outline of what is realistic (even with specialist referral) will be helpful at the initial stage.

- Psychosexual medicine is not foreign territory, and the health professional can use familiar cues from general consultations, for example 'How long?' or 'What do you think is the matter?', or emotional cues from everyday consultations, such as 'How does this problem make you feel?' or 'How is it affecting your relationship(s)?' It is useful to consider why the patient is presenting at this time, especially if the problem is a chronic one. *Has he or she come or was he or she sent, and if so, by whom?*

- The health professional should look for underlying health concerns, as the scenario is often that of the 'straw that broke the camel's back', for example a difficult delivery, the stress of first-time parenthood, plus anaemia leading to low libido. The 'psychosexual problem' is then cured by a sympathetic ear, reassurance and iron tablets.

- A different approach may be needed for a covert presentation of sexual problems. Common covert presentations include fatigue, depression, relationship problems or chronic non-specific gynaecological complaints. A doctor comfortable with a 'sexual relationship' line of questioning may uncover the underlying problem.

- It is worth finding out how the 'problem' is affecting current relationships (or lack thereof), and whether or not it was also an issue in previous relationships. In general, chronic or recurring problems are more likely to need specialist referral. As a rule of thumb, any problem of from two to three months to one year's duration will probably be resolved without referral, but where there is a recurring problem, especially with a change of partner, eventual referral is likely.

- Specific questions should be asked to detect anxiety and depression, and whether or not the patient has any specific concerns about genital health (which may reveal the 'worried well' or real concerns about HIV). This question is particularly useful postnatally, when women may have fantasies of internal damage. The reassurance of an examination and an invitation or permission to inspect the area for themselves can be curative.

- Other useful areas of questioning include:
  - general life-style – this may elicit practical problems such as lack of privacy, exhaustion due to overcommitment, unemployment or work promotion
  - possible unresolved issues around fertility and contraception
  - whether expectations have changed within the relationship or the wider extended family
  - whether the patient has tried any other avenue of professional or self-help
  - whether alcohol or other substance 'misuse' is a problem
  - how the partner is coping. Is he or she part of the problem or part of the solution?

In general, it makes sense for the health professional to deal with issues that he or she would usually accept within the remit of general practice, refer relationship problems to Relate (formerly the Marriage Guidance Council), and refer long-term problems outside his or her expertise to a local specialist. It is essential to approach the patient's problem non-judgementally and with an open mind.

Sexuality is an expression of each person's core identity, and any consensual sexual expression is to be respected. The professional's role is to advise on patients' health and sexual happiness, which promotes physical and mental well-being. It helps to *not assume* that all patients aspire to suburban, able-bodied, heterosexual marriage; that way, one is prepared to look at the patient's agenda.

Even where referral is appropriate, the approach and groundwork of the referring GP can make an enormous difference to the success or failure of specialist intervention. Going to a psychosexual clinic is a daunting experience. Being referred by a doctor who has been helpful and has taken the time to explain the clinic's approach and what the patient can expect may determine whether or not the patient accepts the offer and/or turns up for the appointment.

Some areas of the UK do not have access to specialist clinics and rely on a hotch-potch of psychiatry, gynaecology or urology provision. If this is the case, the GP can ask the FHSA or other service providers who the named specialists are, and then write and ask them to describe their approach and management.

Common presenting problems

Common presenting problems include the following.

Low libido

Clues about general health problems, particularly anaemia and hypothyroidism, should be included in the history. The GP should be prepared to follow up the unusual, since this is such a generalized presentation. Open-ended questions should be used liberally and full blood count (FBC) and thyroid function test (TFT) included in routine tests. Depression is a common covert presentation of low libido.

Dyspareunia or pain on intercourse

History and examination are needed to exclude endometriosis, adenomyosis and pelvic inflammatory disease. Investigations may include high vaginal swab and chlamydial swab (with, if necessary, referral to a GUM clinic for chlamydia testing) and a pelvic ultra-sound scan. Referral for laparoscopy may also be needed.

Again, the history can be open ended, with general questions about fears, anxieties and relationship issues. Is it a new relationship; has the pattern of intercourse changed; is there anything to elicit feelings of guilt (the euphemism 'disquiet' may be less loaded)? The GP should have a higher than usual suspicion of previous sexual abuse in such a case.

Pelvic examination is central to the management of this problem, and it is important to be particularly careful about the 'niceties' of the examination, such as warming the speculum. Male GPs should give consideration to the issue of chaperoning: this is definitely advisable where the presenting problem is psychosexual. The examination should be approached with a view to finding out as much as possible on several different levels:

- *psychological* – for example undue apprehension

- *physical* – is the pain elicited on examination? Is it the same pain, and can the patient describe it? Is the pain described consistent with the extent of the examination and/or pathological considerations? Is there vaginismus?

- *emotional* – deep-rooted emotional problems require specialist resources, but the GP may be in a privileged position of being easily able to refer to the emotional impact of such a distressing complaint. A respectful enquiry while carrying out the examination can be particularly revealing. The focus should be on both verbal and non-verbal reactions.

This type of examination needs time, without the pressure of a queue of waiting patients, so if possible the patient should be asked to come back when this can be arranged. Otherwise, the GP should concentrate on a basic pelvic examination and then proceed with referral as necessary.

Premature ejaculation

The most relevant questions here are those of duration and recurrence. A history lasting less than six to twelve months has a fairly optimistic outlook. Again, psychological precipitating factors should be sought.

If an erection can be maintained during masturbation without premature ejaculation, the patient can be reassured that there is no physical problem. As in the case of dyspareunia, examination allows exploration of worries and anxieties, for example of the 'Am I normal?' variety, especially for young men or the sexually inexperienced. Reassurance can be very beneficial. There are no specific investigations unless the history suggests underlying health problems.

Impotence

Pathological causes need to be ruled out – diabetic neuropathy, peripheral cardiovascular disease and major abdominal surgery are the main considerations. A careful drug history should be taken. Investigations include FBC and follicle-stimulating hormone (FSH), luteinizing hormone (LH), testosterone and prolactin levels.

Enquiry should be made into masturbation and night erections – if there is normal erection and ejaculation on masturbation, the patient can be reassured there is no physical problem. If there is no masturbation, is the main issue one of low libido? Are there mental health or substance 'misuse' issues? Again, even when the history elicits normal function, examination can be revealing and reassurance part of the solution.

Questions about sexual identity

'Am I normal?', 'Am I lesbian/gay/homosexual/bisexual?' – the health professional cannot possibly know the answer to these questions. However, at the simplest level, the professional can point the patient towards a local help line. It takes very low-key enquiries to find out what the real concerns are, for example family, work or meeting people. An accepting, helpful health professional can avert potential problems of isolation and possibly even suicide.

Conclusion

The GP needs to balance a helpful approach to patients' sexual problems with the complexities of general health care and health promotion. It is a difficult balancing act, but that is part of the challenge of general practice.

5

Disabled people and sexual practice

The 1990s have been marked by much activism by disabled people demanding their rights. Bills presented in parliament and disabled 'activists' taking to the streets are an expression of disabled people's wishes to be treated with respect and equality, to have the same rights and expectations as the rest of society. Among those demands is the right to fulfilling sexual relationships.

Disabled people have been and always will be sexual beings. However, in a climate in which sex and disability is taboo, and sexual expression is denied or actively prohibited, disabled people are forced to find their own solutions, often in isolation and with much unnecessary fear.

Disabled youngsters, like any other young people, will want to explore their bodies, will be anxious about sex, and will want to seek advice, information and support. Unhappily, sex education, advice or family planning services are not available to disabled youngsters as they are to non-disabled ones. Not only are premises inaccessible to many disabled people, but also the information on offer is often not appropriate nor in an accessible format, for example on audio-tape or in Braille.

Are disabled people that different?

It should be remembered that while disabled people's bodies may look or function differently from the 'norm', their hopes, dreams and desires will be the same as those of most people seeking advice or support about sex.

The professional may have the medical information and expertise in dealing with a particular impairment, but the disabled person is the expert on his or her own condition. The unique difference of the condition, what is possible and what may be worth trying will only be discovered by open and honest dialogue with the patient. He or she will know the restrictions and limits that govern day-to-day life and should be trusted to experiment sexually to find out what is really possible. Patients may just need the professional's 'blessing' or a few tips to get them started, as they will probably have faced years of 'can't' and 'shouldn't' from well-meaning family, friends and carers.

Moral debates

Whether people with learning difficulties should be 'allowed' to have sex, whether it is 'fair' for people with disabilities to have children, or whether one should pass on a gay switchboard number to a disabled person may present the professional with a moral dilemma. Although there may be practical difficulties to be overcome and arrangements to be made, the disabled person should not be treated any differently from the non-disabled person. It is important to present all the facts at one's disposal, but, at the end of the day, disabled people must be facilitated to make their own choices.

Body image

When television and magazines are full of beautiful bodies, it is not surprising that many disabled people feel embarrassed, awkward and somewhat ashamed about their bodies. Catheters, colostomies or 'unsightly' lumps and bumps can seem insurmountable obstacles to relationship formation and fulfilling sex. However, the expectation that a disabled person is, or can be, a sexual person can in itself be very uplifting. Recommending a book or pamphlet about sex and/or information about a support group may facilitate the development of self-esteem.

Once in a relationship, the knowledge that one is sexually attractive to others can be a major boost to self-esteem.

Social isolation

Lack of access, negative attitudes to disabled people and poverty are the major barriers to meeting others for friendship and more intimate relationships. An understanding of disabled people's position in society will help, and positive suggestions of ways to meet people are what is needed. Singles or youth clubs, support groups, evening or day-time education to pursue hobbies, disability rights groups and dating agencies provide a variety of ways of meeting friends or partners. However, being able to face disappointment is important. It is helpful for the professional to offer an understanding ear, as rejection may be an all-too-common experience for many disabled people.

Advice for people with specific impairments

Spinal cord injury

Following spinal cord injury, one of the main problems is often confidence and the need to reclaim one's body. Bladder and bowel management are a priority when in hospital, and one's genital area can feel like public property. Overcoming this invasion of one's space and becoming familiar and confident with sex will take time and practice, so the professional should encourage patience.

Getting into a comfortable *position* supported by pillows, in a familiar, safe place, will facilitate relaxation. Worrying about un- wanted bowel or bladder activity is best overcome by talking with one's partner and sticking to one's normal routine. Planning for sex may be necessary, so ensuring an empty bowel or bladder before sex should be part of this.

Worries about performance, for example numbness following in- jury, or lack of an erection, are concerns that need thoughtful advice. Talking about sex can be a real turn-on if one cannot feel touch, and careful positioning of mirrors, so that one can see what is happening, may also facilitate sex. It may not be possible to abandon a catheter or leg-bag during sex, and if this is the case and the person finds it a turn-off, he or she can be encouraged to talk with his or her partner, as this may not be an issue for the partner. Advice about experi- menting with clamping off the catheter or strapping it in position may be helpful.

Medical advice about assistance with erections may be needed. Explanations about penile injections or various erection aids, includ- ing penile prosthetic implants, may resolve the problems. A simple leaflet following consultation, and time to think things over, with the address or telephone number of the Spinal Injuries Association and the opportunity to talk to someone in the same situation, will be of great value in allaying anxieties. Ultimately, trial and error will determine what is best for any particular individual.

Arthritis

The most common problems are those of limitation of movement and pain. Sex may be painful if joints are moved beyond their usual range or if unusually heavy weight is borne. Let pain be the guide, and if anything is painful, the patient should stop and try something else.

Sexual activity that causes pain should be avoided, especially during any flare-up in the person's condition. However, sex is not merely sexual intercourse, and much pleasure can be obtained from massage, stroking, gentle touching and masturbation.

Sex aids, such as a vibrator, may assist a person with limited or painful hand movements in giving pleasure to a partner or him or herself.

If sex is planned, it is advisable to take one's usual analgesics half an hour before sexual activity. Experimenting with position to maximize comfort is important and can, in itself, be exciting and fun. Communication with one's partner is vital – having the confidence to say what is painful or uncomfortable, as well as what is pleasurable, is the only way to successful sex. However, most people find it difficult to be open and honest about sex, so the disabled person has to try to overcome this general disinclination to talk. A sexual problem may have nothing to do with arthritis, and the only way to find this out is through talking.

Good communication stemming from *confidence* is vital for a young person with arthritis, or any disability, who is making the first move into adult relationships. Surviving the knocks of adolescence and the rejection of early relationships will require inner strength, support and a good talk giving the encouragement to carry on.

It should be remembered that, although sex in its various forms is important in a relationship, so are trust and honesty, and kisses and cuddles can say a lot. Sex is not all about penetration and should not be goal-oriented. It helps to take time to express oneself and allow tired and stiff joints to rest.

Cardiorespiratory disability

The aim of rehabilitation is to enable the person to function at the highest possible level, physically, emotionally and socially, consistent with her or his impairment.

Adjustment to disability following an acute dramatic illness may be particularly difficult, and both the disabled person and her or his partner will need time to adjust. Frustration, anger, a sense of loss and guilt are all common reactions. Once home, and away from the hospital environment, carers may find managing the patient particularly difficult. Overprotective carers may delay recovery by preventing exercise and restricting activity.

Anxiety about resuming sexual activity is common, but sudden death during sexual intercourse is very rare. Reassurance and encouragement to maintain activity and become more independent will also aid in regaining confidence. The usual advice is to resume sexual activity four to six weeks after a myocardial infarction.

Conclusion

There are far too many forms of impairment to be included in this short chapter, and the above are merely examples – of disability owing to trauma, which is static and ongoing, of a chronic painful impairment, and of a disability resulting from an acute medical condition.

However, whatever the impairment, the approach should be largely the same, encompassing:

- recognition of the disabled person's sexuality

- advice and management of practical issues, where appropriate

- support and encouragement to enable the disabled person to find his or her own solutions.

Self-esteem, confidence in relationships and opportunities in life should not be seen as the preserve of the non-disabled. Primary care professionals are in a prime position to create positive expectations.

6

Contraception provision

Contraception provision is part of the core work of most general practices. However, given the importance of access to appropriate, accurate information and contraceptive supplies for many women, effort spent in enhancing the provision of this service is very worth while. In contraception provision, as in other areas of sexual health, it is important to acknowledge that it is the service user who decides what course to follow. The role of the provider is not to decide, but to inform and support users in taking the best decisions for themselves. Compliance in using contraceptive measures effectively depends on the user making informed, appropriate choices, and then following them through.

This section inevitably reflects the fact that contraception, apart from in relationships in which condoms or male sterilization is used, is largely a task for women. This concentration on the issues for women should be counterbalanced by a perspective that acknowledges that the responsibility for the outcome of sexual behaviour is best shared between the participants.

Providing information within contraceptive services

The essence of good contraceptive practice is information and support for those needing it. This includes three aspects: information to support the choice of provider, the choice of method, and compliance with the chosen method.

Information about the range of methods available at the practice and arrangements for women's health or family planning appointments, including emergency contraception, should be clearly displayed. It is much easier for some people to help themselves to this information than to ask a receptionist or other staff member. Posters and leaflets are also important in signalling the availability and willingness of staff to discuss sexual health, and this will reassure whose who are embarrassed or concerned about tackling their need for contraception.

All contraceptive methods have benefits and costs in health terms and in terms of ease of use and reliability. Many women will use three or more different methods at different stages of their fertile lives. One of the tasks of contraceptive practice is to help women balance risks and benefits to find the best method for their current circumstances. The Family Planning Association has produced a leaflet that compares the advantages and disadvantages of currently available methods. In contrast, information supplied by manufacturers tends to reflect their own products, rather than being a comparison across the full range of methods.

Many doctors underestimate the importance of providing written information to back up discussion about compliance 'rules' for using and staying safe with a particular contraceptive method. There is no substitute for providing adequate time to explore and explain the mode of action of the chosen method and how to use it for maximum effectiveness, and to answer questions. However, it does not take much further time to say that basic information about the method is contained in a leaflet that the patient can take home, and to encourage the patient to return with any queries or problems.

Despite strenuous efforts, consistent advice has still not been agreed for women using combined oral contraceptives who miss tablets or whose protection is otherwise decreased (for example because of a drug interaction or severe diarrhoea). It is important to check that everyone in the practice is teaching the same set of 'pill rules', and that patients are warned if these differ from advice in the pill packet inserts. In these circumstances, it is particularly important to provide written material to back up oral instruction.

Most decisions about sexual behaviour are made without consulting a health professional, and many people have difficulty in seeking health care with regard to potentially difficult and embarrassing issues surrounding sexuality. However, for most contraceptive methods, clinical consultation is necessary to obtain supplies, as are further visits for check-ups and repeat supplies. Health professionals are thus in the delicate position of trying to provide services that people will use to stay well, without medicalizing one of the most personal and intimate areas of human life. It is often at times of crisis and change that contraceptive problems become acute and patients find it hardest to acknowledge and secure the help they need, for example for post-coital contraception.

How the practice is organized is important in enabling patients to get the best possible care.

- Some patients welcome the chance of booking into a general surgery session for contraception because they feel that then no-one else will know why they are attending.

- Others prefer to attend designated Well Woman/family planning appointments where they know they will have 'more specialized' attention.

- Arrangements are needed to ensure that there is time during each working day to see women requiring post-coital contraception. Many people do not know that post-coital methods do not have to be used as soon as 'the morning after', and this greatly raises the anxiety of patients needing to be seen. Sensitivity is needed from all the practice team to enable women to be seen within the time limits (72 hours after intercourse for the oral method, five days for an IUCD) without their feeling they have to explain their hurry in a way that feels difficult.

- It takes longer than a standard appointment time to discuss different contraceptive methods, help the patient to make the best choice, and teach the use of the chosen method. Competing demands have therefore to be reconciled when dealing with patients who present with contraceptive problems in standard surgeries.

- It helps if all practice staff agree consistent standards, for example a limited list of preferred contraceptives, an outline of history-taking for contraception, information materials for service users, and a shared understanding of confidentiality as it applies to contraceptive care.

Family planning history

General medical history

- Current illness, including current medication
- Relevant family history (including breast cancer and diabetes)
- Risk factors for cardiovascular disease
- Any previous adverse reactions to medicines

Gynaecological history

- Age at menarche
- Age at first sexual intercourse
- Previous and current sexual relationships
- Any pregnancies and their outcome
- Plans for future pregnancies
- Pattern of menstruation – previous /current:
    - duration of bleeding
    - frequency of bleeding
    - amount of bleeding .
- Presence of:
    - dysmenorrhoea
    - intermenstrual bleeding
    - premenstrual symptoms
    - vaginal discharge
    - urinary symptoms

Contraceptive history

- Previous contraceptive methods used and outcomes

- Duration of total accumulated combined oral contraceptive use

Screening checks

- Cervical cytology

- Rubella antibody status

- Sickle-cell screening

Figures suggest that only about one-third of sexually active women under the age of 16 are seen in family planning clinics outside general practice. No comparable figures are available for general practice, but there are probably a large number of sexually active young people who are not in contact with any professional source of advice about contraception. Given that very young pregnancies carry a high risk of poor health and/or social outcome for mother and baby, young people who decide to have a sexual relationship before being in a position to undertake the responsibilities of parenthood need access to caring and professional advice and measures to minimize risks to their health and future fertility. However, sexually active under-16-year-olds are often concerned that GPs and practice staff will not respect their confidentiality. They may mistakenly believe that GPs are legally obliged to inform their parents if they request contraception. It is important to provide information to ensure that young people understand the confidentiality they can expect.

Consultations about contraception may be the only chance that many women have of asking questions and airing their concerns about menstruation, fertility and the mechanics of sexuality. The specialized family planning services have developed a *pro forma* history (see box) that enables the professional to form a picture of the individual woman's feelings and responses to her menstrual cycle, sexual activity, current and past sexual relationships and fertility, in order to provide the best advice for the individual. When taking such a history at a first interview, it may not always be appropriate to discuss risk factors for STDs and HIV and the use of condoms in detail, especially if the main concern is the risk of unplanned pregnancy. However, helping the patient to understand how her and her partner(s)' sexual behaviour and choice of contraceptive strategy may influence STD risks can be included either at the first visit or on reviewing the history at a subsequent visit, as appropriate, and recorded in the notes.

Family planning methods and prevention of STDs and HIV

Interactions between family planning methods and STD/HIV prevention can be summarized as follows. In comparing different methods it is important to take into account that:

* for most methods, effectiveness depends on the user and his or her partner

* methods vary as to who is *in control* of their use

* the appropriateness of a particular method depends partly on the nature of the relationship(s) in which it is to be used

* the male condom and the female condom (placed over the penis with the inner ring removed) can be used to reduce the risk of transmission of infections through anal intercourse between heterosexual or homosexual partners.

The male condom

* Efficiency against pregnancy: 85–98% in different studies with different populations.

* How it works: Prevents sperm from entering the vagina.

* Pros: Good barrier against infection. Protects against cervical cancer.

* Cons: Must put on erect penis. May slip off or split. Man needs to withdraw after ejaculation. New condom must be used each time. Oil-based lubricants should not be used – they may damage the condom.

* Problems/protection against STDs: Can offer total protection against STDs. Studies vary – protection against *Neisseria gonorrhoeae* said to be 20–100%, but there are problems as

some studies are self-reported or retrospective. In vitro, there is total protection against chlamydia, herpes simplex, cytomegalovirus and gonoccocus.

- Problems/protection against HIV: In vitro, total protection. Out of the laboratory it appears to give good, but not total, protection against HIV. Protects against reinfection/cross-infection if one or both partners is HIV positive. (There is some theoretical evidence that reinfection may increase the rate of progression to AIDS.)

The female condom

- Efficiency against pregnancy: 93–98% (in small studies among stable couples who were previously regular users of condoms or caps). No large-scale studies have been carried out.

- How it works: Barrier against sperm (and organisms).

- Pros: Can be put in before sex. Protects against cervical cancer. Oil-based products can be used.

- Cons: Penis must enter the condom, rather than pass into the vagina outside the condom. May slip. Expensive.

- Problems/protection against STDs: Protects against all infections. Early (only small-scale) studies show better protection than with the male condom.

- Problems/protection against HIV: Protects against HIV, as for male condom.

Natural methods

- Efficiency against pregnancy: 80–98%.

- How it works: Avoid intercourse at fertile time.

- Pros: No side-effects. No products needed. Woman aware of her body cycle.

- Cons: Unable to use if there are irregular periods or after having a baby. Requires negotiation between partners.

* Problems/protection against STDs: No protection.

* Problems/protection against HIV: No protection.

Diaphragm/cervical cap

* Efficiency against pregnancy: 85–96%.

* How it works: Acts as a barrier against sperm entering the uterus.

* Pros: Protects against cervical cancer. Use only when needed.

* Cons: Need to use each time and leave for six hours post-intercourse. If inserted more than three hours beforehand, extra spermicide is required. Need to refit each year, if weight changes and postnatally.

* Problems/protection against STDs: Some protection against STDs. Reduced rates of gonococcal cervicitis, less hospitalization for pelvic inflammatory disease. May be better for women than the condom because of the use of spermicide. Reduced cervical pre-cancerous changes.

* Problems/protection against HIV: No evidence of barrier against HIV.

Spermicides (usually nonoxynol-9)

* Efficiency against pregnancy: Used alone, 75%. With cap, 90–98%.

* How it works: Kills sperm.

* Problems/protection against STDs: Kills all common STD infections in vitro. Modifies vaginal flora, leading to an increased risk of candida. Heavy users may get vaginitis and minor ulceration, increasing the risk of STD.

* Problems/protection against HIV: Antiviral in vitro. Not proven in vivo. As with STDs, the risk of ulceration, especially of the anus, may increase HIV risk.

Combined oral contraceptive pill (COC)

* Efficiency against pregnancy: 97–99%.

* How it works: Contains oestrogen and progestogen. Stops ovulation. Thickens cervical mucus.

- Pros: Easy. Effective. No interference with sex. Reduced period pains and PMT. Protects against cancer of the ovary and uterus.

- Cons: Increased risk of cervical changes and cancer. Alters drugs that pass through liver. Increased risk of hypertension. Affects mucosa. Possible increase in incidence of cancer of liver and breast. Increased risk of gallstones.

- Problems/protection against STDs: No protection against STD infections. Alters mucosa, possibly encouraging infection.

- Problems/protection against HIV: May be immunosuppressive in HIV-negative women; the significance of this for HIV-positive women is unclear. No protection against HIV.

Progestogen-only pill (POP)

- Efficiency against pregnancy: 96–99%.

- How it works: Makes mucosa hostile to sperm and womb hostile to egg. May stop ovulation.

- Pros: Easy (except very small margin of error). No interference with sex. No link with cardiovascular disease. Can be used when breast-feeding.

- Cons: Irregular or no periods. Needs to be taken within three hours of same time each day. Reduced efficiency in women over 70 kg in weight. Increased risk of ectopic pregnancy.

- Problems/protection against STDs: No protection. Need to combine with condom.

- Problems/protection against HIV: No protection. Reduces the amount of blood loss, which is useful in HIV-positive women.

Injectable contraception

- Efficiency against pregnancy: 99%.

- How it works: Stops ovulation.

- Pros: No interference with sex. Protects against cancer of the uterus. Lasts three months (Depo-Provera) or two months (Noristerat).

- Cons: Irregular periods. If side-effects unacceptable, cannot be taken out. Reduced fertility for one year afterwards. ?increased weight. ?increased depression.

- Problems/protection against STDs: No protection.

- Problems/protection against HIV: No protection. Useful in HIV-positive women because of reduced blood loss.

Implant (Norplant)

- Efficiency against pregnancy: First year 99%, two to five years 98%.

- How it works: Releases progestogen, which prevents egg and sperm meeting. Reduces ovulation.

- Pros: No interference with sex. Lasts for five years. Fertility restored when removed.

- Cons: Irregular periods, especially in the first year, plus inter-menstrual bleeding. Headache, acne, nausea, breast tenderness and increased weight.

- Problems/protection against STDs: No protection.

- Problems/protection against HIV: Reduced blood loss. Combine with condom.

Emergency contraception – pill

- Efficiency against pregnancy: 96–99%.

- How it works: Alters hormone balance.

- Pros: Use within 72 hours of intercourse.

- Cons: Nausea and vomiting.

- Problems/protection against STDs: No protection.

- Problems/protection against HIV: No protection.

Emergency contraception – IUCD

- Efficiency against pregnancy: 99%.

- How it works: Acts as a foreign body and prevents implantation.

- Pros: Use within five days of intercourse. Ongoing method.

- Cons: Risk of pelvic inflammatory disease.

- Problems/protection against STDs: No protection.

- Problems/protection against HIV: No protection.

Intrauterine contraceptive device (IUCD)

- Efficiency against pregnancy: 98–99%.

- How it works: Impairs the viability of egg and sperm. Prevents egg and sperm meeting, and prevents implantation.

- Pros: Works immediately and lasts for at least five years. No interference with sex. Previously, IUCDs gave no protection against ectopic pregnancy. Now, with the use of copper, the risk of an ectopic is reduced to one-tenth of that for no contraception. New progestogen-releasing devices may be available, which reduce menstrual loss and work for at least three years.

- Cons: Risk of pelvic inflammatory disease, leading to risk of infertility. Increased blood loss (non-progestogen-releasing IUCDs). Not to be used in primigravidae because of the risk of pelvic inflammatory disease. Uterine perforation (increased risk in post-natal and [possibly] lactating women).

- Problems/protection against STDs: No protection, and probably increase risk. Chlamydia should be screened for before insertion. Increased risk in women with multiple partners. Newer IUCDs show improvements in pelvic inflammatory disease rates (the copper T has a rate of pelvic inflammatory disease per 100 women after one year of 2.9%, but reduces with subsequent years).

- Problems/protection against HIV: No protection, and possible increased risk because of increased blood loss (non-progestogen-releasing IUCDS). Not be used in HIV-positive women because of increased blood loss, leading to anaemia, risk of pelvic inflammatory disease and risk of actinomyces infection, which may be lethal in HIV.

Sponge

- Efficiency against pregnancy: 75–90%?

- How it works: Barrier method. Traps vaginal and seminal fluid. Also has a spermicide (nonoxynol-9) incorporated.

- Pros: Works for 24 hours, during which the woman can have sex more than once.

- Cons: Expensive. Unreliable. Cannot be used during periods.

- Problems/protection against STDs: May offer some protection.

- Problems/protection against HIV: Not known. Not recommended.

Female sterilization

- Efficiency against pregnancy: 99+%.

- How it works: The fallopian tube is cut, so that the egg does not reach the sperm.

- Pros: Permanent. Effective immediately postoperatively. No interference with sex.

- Cons: Permanent. Pelvic inflammatory disease has been noted.

- Problems/protection against STDs: No protection. Use with condom.

- Problems/protection against HIV: No protection. Use with condom.

Male sterilization

- Efficiency against pregnancy: 99+%.

- How it works: Vas deferens is cut. No sperm appear in seminal fluid.

- Pros: Permanent. No interference with intercourse.

- Cons: Need to check a few months postoperatively that all sperm are gone. May be an increased risk of kidney stones, prostate cancer and testicular cancer.

- Problems/protection against STDs: No protection.

- Problems/protection against HIV: No protection. Use with condom.

7

Management of sexually transmitted diseases

Sexually transmitted diseases are common and, if inadequately treated, can have serious long-term sequelae. In women, these may include pelvic pain, infertility and ectopic pregnancy; men may develop arthropathy or iritis. In big cities, many patients who think they have an STD are likely to attend the local GUM clinic, but in many other areas the GUM service is patchy or inadequate, with clinics that are poorly advertised or offer a limited service. In these areas, the GP may be the first port of call, and, even in London, patients may consult their GP, not realizing that their symptoms are due to an STD. Some patients may prefer to visit the GP, and it can be difficult to persuade them to attend a GUM clinic. For these reasons, all GPs need a working understanding of the diagnosis, investigation and management of the common STDs.

The following section describes the common presentations in men and women separately.

Women

Women often present with vaginal discharge. This may be physiological or pathological, and the history will go some way towards distinguishing between these alternatives. A physiological discharge is usually clear and odourless, and may be more profuse mid-cycle.

Candida

The area is typically itchy, white and sore. The condition is very common. Genitourinary physicians find a co-existent STD in 30% of women with thrush; although this finding is unlikely to be replicated in a general practice population, it is worth considering the possibility. A high vaginal swab will confirm the presence of candida, and an endocervical swab for chlamydia can be taken at the same time. Treatment should be with topical antifungals (e.g. clotrimazole pessaries) or, if necessary, oral triazoles (e.g. fluconazole 150 mg as a single oral dose).

Recurrent candidiasis can be difficult to treat. Diabetes or causes of immune deficiency should first be excluded. The diagnosis should be checked by high vaginal and endocervical swabbing. It is often worth treating both partners for two to four weeks: women with clotrimazole pessaries 200 mg nightly and clotrimazole 1% cream, men with clotrimazole cream to use under the foreskin twice daily. If this fails, referral to a GUM clinic should be considered, both to verify the diagnosis and to exclude co-existent infection.

Anaerobic vaginosis (Gardnerella, bacterial vaginosis)

Typically there is a fishy odour, and often a yellowy discharge. Anaerobic vaginosis may be implicated in premature labour. Women often mistake this condition for thrush, but the diagnosis is easy to make in general practice because the vaginal secretions lose their usual acidity. Placing some discharge on pH paper will quickly confirm the diagnosis – the normal pH of the vagina is about 4, whereas in anaerobic vaginosis it rises to 6 or 7. A high vaginal swab may reveal clue cells. This condition is not necessarily sexually transmitted, and is best described to women as an imbalance of the normal flora in the vagina. The 'good' bacteria that maintain the acidity of the vagina have been replaced with 'bad' ones, which prevent the 'good' ones growing. Oral metronidazole 2 g as a single dose kills the anaerobes, which usually allows the lactobacilli to re-establish. Occasionally, Aci-Jel is useful to maintain the vaginal pH while the normal flora re-establishes itself.

Trichomonas vaginalis

The incubation period is one to three weeks. There is often an offensive, frothy, yellowy-green discharge, although the infection can be asymptomatic. It is difficult to diagnose in general practice as a special culture medium is required. Treatment is with metronidazole 2 g as a single dose, treating sexual partners at the same time.

Chlamydia

This is an important cause of morbidity in women, as it can lead to pelvic inflammatory disease and the ensuing complications of pelvic pain, infertility and ectopic pregnancy. It is often asymptomatic in women. Contact tracing is vital.

Chlamydia should be considered in women with vaginal discharge, intermenstrual or post-coital bleeding, dyspareunia, dysmenorrhoea/ menorrhagia or pelvic pain. Recent studies have found a prevalence of chlamydia of 8% in women requesting termination of pregnancy and in women having symptoms requiring speculum investigation. Women who swab positive for chlamydia have a 60% likelihood of developing pelvic infection post-termination of pregnancy, which is a good argument for swabbing and, where appropriate, treating all women prior to the termination. The easiest method of detecting chlamydia in general practice is enzyme immunoassay (EIA). This requires special chlamydia swabs, which need to be taken from the endocervix. First, the cervix should be wiped clean, and then the swab inserted well into the endocervix and rotated vigorously. Ideally, a urethral swab should be taken at the same time, as this will identify approximately 20–30% of women not detected from endo-cervical swabs alone.

Treatment is with doxycycline 100 mg twice daily for seven days, or with erythromycin 1 g twice daily for 14 days, or with the new drug azithromycin 1 g as a single dose. Contact tracing is mandatory; as this can be difficult in general practice, it may require referral to a GUM clinic.

Gonorrhoea

The incubation period is three to five days. Gonorrhoea is not often seen in general practice, but it can cause severe acute pelvic in-flammatory disease with purulent cervical discharge and severe dysuria ('peeing broken glass'). It may be asymptomatic in women. The infection is best dealt with in a specialist clinic, as test of cure and contact tracing are needed. In an emergency, treatment should be with a single dose either of amoxycillin 3 g + probenecid 1 g, or of ciprofloxacin 250 mg. The likelihood of concomitant chlamydial infection is extremely high, so patients should also have a course of doxycycline, as above.

Syphilis

GUM clinics check all attending patients for syphilis serology. This blanket approach is at odds with the GP problem-oriented approach, and is unlikely to find favour with GPs. If syphilis is suspected, blood should be taken for serology; if the result is positive, the patient should be referred.

Men

Men are much more likely to go to a GUM clinic than a GP if they notice urethral discharge or dysuria; it is also usually relatively easy to persuade men to attend a GUM clinic. This is to be encouraged, as GUM clinics are able to make on-the-spot diagnoses from microscopic examination of secretions obtained from urethral swabs, as well as obtaining microbiological confirmation. Moreover, GUM clinics will routinely test for all STDs, since many patients will have more than one infection. Thus, a man with urethral discharge or dysuria and a negative midstream urine sample (MSU) should be referred. Men may also present to their GP with scabies or 'crabs' (pubic lice). Although these can easily be treated in general practice with the appropriate parasiticidal preparations, there may well be a co-existing STD, and careful history-taking is necessary.

Treatment of partners

It makes no sense to treat a person for an STD and not treat his or her sexual partner(s). If the partner(s) cannot be persuaded to go to a GUM clinic, both the index patient and the sexual partner(s) should be treated by the GP, and asked to refrain from sexual intercourse until treatment is completed. GUM clinics usually do a test of cure before allowing couples to recommence sexual activity. The exception is chlamydia, which is so sensitive to doxycycline that test of cure is not considered necessary if the patient has completed the course of antibiotics.

8

Liaison and support services

Genitourinary medicine and family planning services

There are few parts of the NHS in which it is commonly understood that 'It's OK to talk about sex here'. GUM and family planning clinics outside general practice are self-referral services that specifically offer a degree of anonymity and a choice of provider, with the aim of ensuring that all who need these services can find an easily accessible, free and confidential provider whom they are prepared to use.

However, most 'sexual health' consultations, especially those concerning contraception, happen in general practice. This highlights the importance of effective interactions and working links between the three key providers: general practices, GUM clinics and family planning clinics.

The rationale for continuing open access to GUM and family planning clinics is to provide patients with further choice, recognizing that sexual health raises sensitive issues and that encouraging take-up of these services benefits the public health as well as the health of the individuals concerned, in terms of controlling the spread of STDs and unplanned conception rates. So, how successful have GUM and family planning services been?

- While the perceived need to maintain absolute confidentiality has provided an important reassurance for patients, it has often meant relative isolation from other services, seen, for example, in the reluctance of many GUM clinics to communicate with GPs.

- Ease of access can be difficult to achieve. Although most services are 'open access', in that patients can self-refer, many are little publicized, open at inconvenient times and/or difficult to locate. These factors tend to perpetuate the aura of secretiveness associated with sexual health.

- Patients using these services enjoy the ready availability of advice and expertise, the range of contraceptive methods on offer, the relative immediacy of diagnosis and treatment, and the fact that medication is free. Some patients attend these services to obtain a 'second opinion' or a means of gaining access to other hospital-based specialties, such as gynaecology, although this has implications for funding arrangements.

The goal of improving liaison between services obviously requires flexibility and goodwill on all sides, rather than the apportioning of blame for past and current problems, where these exist. From the general practice perspective, it is important to recognize the added value that alternative service providers offer for some patients. For example, many young people who attend specialist family planning services do so because they see their GP as a 'family doctor' who is particularly closely identified with their home situation. Insofar as establishing personal responsibility for one's sexual life involves finding areas of intimacy outside one's family of origin, it is not surprising that, despite liking and respecting their 'family doctor', many young people prefer an alternative professional's advice about this area of their lives.

Steps that general practitioners can take to improve liaison include:

- giving information about GUM and specialist family planning services alongside services offered by the practice itself, in practice leaflets, posters etc.

- developing practice protocols on referral, including requesting discharge information and offering to participate in follow-up (subject to the patient's consent)

- it is also worth remembering that patients can attend a general practice other than the one where they are registered specifically for family planning services. Especially if specialist family planning clinics are not readily accessible locally, it may be helpful for the practice to indicate that it is prepared to see non-registered patients for this purpose.

Potential benefits of closer working relationships between service providers

Opportunities to develop joint management protocols and guidelines, including criteria for referral between services. Possible topics for guidelines include:

- routine contraception

- contraception for special groups, for example HIV-positive women, young people and sex workers

- emergency contraception

- pregnancy counselling and termination of pregnancy

- sexually transmitted infections

- non-sexually transmitted genitourinary conditions, for example candidiasis, cystitis and bacterial vaginosis

- management of sexual assault

- sexual dysfunction.

Potential benefits include:

- improved management for individual patients – ensuring that important signs and symptoms are recognized, early referrals made when appropriate and necessary tests performed for accurate early diagnosis, and ensuring continuity of care and the ready availability of appropriate treatment and advice

- reduction in the spread of STDs and HIV through earlier referral, diagnosis and treatment

- earlier recognition of inadequate contraception and strategies for what to do about it, leading to fewer unwanted conceptions

- streamlined services for termination of pregnancy, leading to fewer late terminations

- destigmatization of sexual health and sexually transmitted infections

- cost savings from avoidance of repeated courses of unnecessary or inappropriate empirical treatments and duplication of tests such as cervical smears

- scope for developing innovative models of joint care for 'problem' conditions, for example recurrent bacterial vaginosis, chronic candidiasis and chronic prostatitis

- enhanced educational opportunities for staff

- scope for collaborative research projects and joint audit

A more comprehensive approach to improving liaison would be through a local co-ordinating group, involving GPs, practice nurses, family planning and GUM staff, and possibly others, such as FHSA and health authority representatives, primary care facilitators and health promotion staff. The initiative to form such a group might come from any of the key players involved, and the group could then identify and work together on local priority issues, which may include the following.

- Producing a local sexual health services directory (and brief leaflets for patients covering the main open-access services), giving details such as:

    - opening times

    - site, accessibility, telephone and fax numbers

    - the referral procedure

    - a description of the services provided and relevant personnel

    - the availability of results and follow-up arrangements

    - what patients can expect on their first visit

    for services including:

    - GUM

- specialist family planning clinics

- specialist young people's clinics and services, for example Brook Advisory Centres

- termination of pregnancy

- psychosexual counselling

- sterilization of women and men

- antenatal care and genetic counselling

• Seeking agreement on local operational matters such as:

- referral criteria and management guidelines for common conditions

- mechanisms for feedback and communication between services

- policies for handling test results (e.g. smears)

- policies on tertiary referrals from GUM and specialist family planning clinics to other specialties, especially for fund holders' patients.

• Organizing joint educational meetings, case presentations, collaborative research and audit.

• Agreeing local outcome targets. Possible indicators might include:

- reducing the number of women presenting for termination of pregnancy by each stage of gestation

- increasing the proportion of women screened for STDs prior to termination of pregnancy

- reducing the incidence of gonorrhoea reinfection

- reducing the incidence of chlamydial infection

- reducing the time from presentation to definitive diagnosis for women with vaginal discharge and men with urethral symptoms

- increasing the proportion of women with inflammatory smears screened for STDs

- increasing the uptake of hepatitis B vaccine in 'at risk' groups, including medical and nursing staff.

• The idea of bringing GUM clinics into general practice is an interesting one that has yet to be explored. As well as benefits, there are potential drawbacks:

  - the loss of anonymity for patients

  - the acute nature of many STDs, which is not readily amenable to a clinic booked in advance

  - the problem of making an accurate 'on the spot' diagnosis without the necessary equipment.

New factors coming into operation that are likely to alter established relationships between general practice, GUM and family planning

• Changes in funding and contracting arrangements

• Pressures to steer resources from hospital-based services into primary health care

• The development of community gynaecology services

• Improving facilities in general practice

• The expanding roles of nurse practitioners

• Developing patterns of 'shared care', for example for patients with HIV disease

---

Drugs services

Detailed discussion of the management of drug-using patients is beyond the scope of this publication, but good liaison between services can be important in ensuring that the general and sexual health needs of drug users are not neglected. Official strategies for tackling drug misuse place increasing emphasis on multiagency and collaborative working, for example involving the police, education and youth services, as well as health authorities. Following a recent government White Paper, each district health authority is being asked to set up a high-level Drug Action Team to promote liaison between NHS, local authority, education, police, prison and probation services. These teams will be advised by multidisciplinary Drug Reference Groups, which should include representation from general practice, via the Local Medical Committee, and which will draw together all interested parties, including voluntary and community organizations, social services, community pharmacy, specialist HIV and drug services, health promotion and business interests. In some districts, similar arrangements already exist.

In addition, the Department of Health is asking health authorities to review arrangements for sharing the care of drug users between specialist providers (including voluntary organizations) and primary care, and to improve access to information about treatment services. This may be an opportunity to improve liaison and clarify the roles of different services. Further changes may be expected after the report of the Department's task force on the effectiveness of treatment services for drug misusers is published in 1996.

Primary care facilitators

In some areas, facilitators for HIV/AIDS and/or sexual health have been appointed, mostly by FHSAs, to support primary health care teams in developing their services, and such appointments may be under consideration in other areas. There is some debate about how well this model of facilitation, which was originally developed for arterial disease prevention, transfers to sexual health, but there is little doubt that a facilitator can provide some useful services. The role of facilitators should be just what the name suggests – not to be an expert but to help practices to recognize and respond to the challenges of sexual health promotion. Among the ways in which facilitators can help are:

- supporting and advising practice teams to develop practice policies and protocols for sexual health promotion

- enabling practice teams to keep abreast of new knowledge, relevant data (e.g. local teenage pregnancy rates compared to

national ones) and examples of good practice culled from local
and national sources by:

- – fostering links with relevant agencies and workers, for example
  through GP/practice nurse/practice manager groups

- – producing regular newsletters or fact sheets

• helping practices to clarify what they are able and willing to
  undertake in the field of sexual health, given other work-loads

• keeping practice teams informed about locally and nationally
  available services and resources, for example the support offered
  by health promotion units, that can help them.

• assessing training needs for all members of the primary health
  care team, and organizing training with PGEA and, if possible,
  academic accreditation for nurses

• developing links between general practice and other services,
  for example by undertaking a liaison role and organizing joint
  seminars and interagency meetings

• organizing and evaluating pilot projects and conducting research.

The appointment of a facilitator is not a panacea that will enable GPs
and nurses effortlessly to develop effective sexual health promotion
services. Ideally, there should be consultation with primary care
teams and other interested parties before a facilitator is appointed,
and the following issues should be addressed.

• What are the aims and priorities for the facilitator's work? Given
  that funding for the post is likely to be short term, a clear job
  description that sets realistic expectations and time-scales is
  needed.

• Since facilitation evolves gradually through the establishment of
  relationships and credibility, what will happen beyond the initial
  life of the project? Is there a commitment on the part of the FHSA
  or commissioning authority to maintain activities such as training
  courses, and to translate findings into service developments?

• What structured support and supervision will the facilitator
  have? Peer support, line management, an advisory group com-
  prising primary care professionals and an appraisal system are all
  needed.

- Will the role of the facilitator be evaluated, and, if so, how?

- What incentives will the facilitator have to offer to motivate primary health care professionals? For example, will there be funds to run courses and provide locum cover to meet identified training needs?

Health promotion departments

Most districts have a health promotion department, which may be part of a larger provider unit, for example community health services. Local arrangements vary as to how the public health function of the purchasing authority fits with the health promotion department, but health promotion departments often have an agency role, commissioning work from a variety of providers, as well as doing it themselves. As district health authorities and FHSAs merge, health promotion departments may take on a greater importance for primary care, for example by taking over responsibility for facilitators. Possible ways in which health promotion departments can support primary care teams include:

- providing training, and organizing conferences and workshops

- facilitating liaison between different sectors, for example by convening local sexual health fora and advisory groups

- offering expert advice and disseminating information, for example about local and national research findings on good practice in health promotion, and on the epidemiology of HIV, STDs and unplanned pregnancy

- commissioning new initiatives, needs assessments, research and audit projects, whether conducted by outsiders to support developments in general practice or by practice teams themselves

- providing posters, leaflets, condoms etc.

There is usually a specific person to contact for advice on sexual health promotion, called a sexual health co-ordinator or an HIV prevention co-ordinator. He or she may be found either on the district health authority purchasing side, usually within the public health team, or

in the health promotion department. With the advent of health com-
missions, sexual health co-ordinators and health promotion departments will potentially play a greater role in supporting general
practice teams in their work. However, in some districts, this may
require active demand from health professionals.

Voluntary services

There are numerous national and local voluntary organizations working in the fields of sexual health, HIV/AIDS and community development, which often has a health component. Typical voluntary
sector activities related to sexual health include:

• mutual support for people with specific conditions such as HIV
  infection, fertility problems, hepatitis B, herpes etc.

• advocacy, lobbying, networking and information exchange

• providing training for professionals and for peer educators,
  volunteers or lay workers

• awareness-raising and health promotion for the general public or
  for specific groups, such as gay men, young people and drug
  users, through events and workshops, producing and distributing
  leaflets, posters and condoms, theatre-in-education, needle exchanges, drop-in centres etc.

• social care provision, for example for people who have AIDS.
  Some voluntary organizations also provide health services, such
  as on-the-spot primary care in drop-in centres and needle exchanges, and hospice or palliative care

• legal and welfare rights advice.

There are clearly many opportunities for members of the general
practice team to work with voluntary organizations – by referring
clients, advertising voluntary sector services in the waiting room,
using literature produced by voluntary organizations, carrying out
clinical sessions as volunteers, serving on boards of management or
medical/nursing advisory panels and using voluntary organizations'
training services. Good relationships with local voluntary organizations may be important in promoting a general practice's image as

being user-friendly and accepting towards groups such as gay men or drug users, since information tends to spread by word of mouth. Equally, good communication can help to prevent awkward situations resulting from misunderstandings about the role of general practice, for example unnecessary requests for people to be seen at practices where they are not registered.

The National AIDS Manual, which is updated regularly from a comprehensive database of (voluntary, statutory and private) services related to HIV/AIDS, is a good source of information about local voluntary organizations. It is rather expensive for most practices to buy, but local health promotion departments may have a copy available for browsing, or the BMA Foundation for AIDS (Tel: 0171 383 6345/6315) can provide information drawn from the manual.

Schools

Primary care professionals often rightly regard school-based sex education (often forming part of personal, social and health education, referred to as PSE or PSHE) as one of the most important elements in teaching young people about sexual health and enabling them to develop the capacity to form healthy, rewarding and responsible sexual relationships. The legal framework for sex education in England and Wales has recently changed, and is as follows.

- In all state schools, the governing body must produce a written policy on sex education.

- Parents have a right to withdraw their children from sex education, where this falls outside the national curriculum.

- At primary and secondary levels, some sexual and reproductive biology is taught in the national curriculum, and is compulsory for all pupils. Parents cannot withdraw children from this.

- At secondary level, schools must provide a wider programme of sex education, which goes beyond the national curriculum and must include HIV/AIDS and STDs.

- At primary level, it is for the governors to decide whether or not to provide a wider programme of sex education, although it is good practice to do so.

• Sex education must, as far as is reasonably practical, be taught in a manner that encourages due regard for moral considerations and the value of family life.

Primary health care teams can support school sex education in various ways.

• They can act as advocates for the importance of sex education and the need for teachers to be trained to deliver it. School governors are key players in this. Purchasers, health promotion and local education authority contacts can also be encouraged to provide support and advice to schools.

• Primary care teams can research and disseminate results about young people's sex education needs, for example, what do girls seeking contraception or abortion say about the teaching they have received?

• Doctors or nurses may be invited into the school to give a talk to pupils on some aspects of sex education. However, this is often not the most effective approach, as health professionals are rarely trained in effective teaching methods for groups of young people. In some cases, inviting a health professional may be a 'soft option', which lets schools off the hook for not developing a properly co-ordinated programme of sex education. Key questions to ask before agreeing to go into a school to teach pupils directly include:

  – What does the school's overall programme of sex education consist of, and how is the health professional's contribution intended to fit within it?

  – What is the school's policy and framework of moral values for sex education? This must be complied with.

  – What material is the health professional expected to cover? How has this been decided upon?

  – What format is envisaged, for example the age and number of pupils, whether a teacher will be present, the time available, whether it is a formal lecture or an open discussion or a question and answer session, and whether or not individual pupils will be able to raise personal concerns in confidence.

How HIV and GUM services are commissioned

As self-referral services for which there is a public health interest in encouraging patients to come forward, the arrangements for commissioning family planning, HIV and GUM services need special consideration. Funding and commissioning arrangements for HIV and GUM services are intended to recognize the importance of ensuring that patients can use these services confidentially, without requiring referral from a GP. However, GPs may still have a role in influencing the commissioning of these services. At the time of writing (1994/95 financial year), the arrangements for England are essentially as follows.

- Health authorities receive specific allocations of funds with which to purchase HIV/AIDS treatment and care. The amount, totalling £164.3 million in 1994/95, is distributed on the basis of a rough measure of case-load (which varies greatly across the country). Although this allocation is separately identified within the authority's budget, it is not ring-fenced, and authorities can decide on the actual amount to spend on HIV/AIDS treatment and care to meet local needs.

- In most areas, the main method of commissioning HIV/AIDS treatment and care is by means of a block contract between a host purchasing authority and a provider unit, such as a GUM department or specialist HIV clinic.

- Health authorities receive an additional allocation with which to commission HIV prevention work, training, HIV counselling and testing, and some GUM and related services. This allocation, totalling £47.6 million in 1994/95, is ring-fenced and must be spent only on the specified HIV-related activities for which it is intended.

- Health authorities are required by law to report annually to the Department of Health on the services they have commissioned for HIV/AIDS prevention, treatment and care, and on numbers of patients treated locally. These reports are intended as a form of performance measurement tool to enable the Department of Health to monitor local service provision.

The implications of these arrangements for primary care may include
those listed below.

• Subject to some exceptions (e.g. hospice care), HIV/AIDS and
  GUM services are open access. Patients can go to the provider of
  their choice without GP referral, and GPs can refer patients to
  any provider.

• Health authorities can commission services from any provider,
  and providers can subcontract to other providers for certain
  services. Authorities are encouraged to consider funding primary
  care prevention work in alliance with FHSAs. This means that
  general practices may be able to get funds for sexual health
  initiatives from FHSAs, from health authorities or from health
  promotion units to whom prevention budgets may be devolved.

• Similarly, where general practices incur costs for treating patients
  with HIV/AIDS (e.g. for prescribing expensive drugs) that go
  beyond what it would be reasonable for the ordinary practice
  budget to bear, there may be a possibility of seeking reimbursement from the health authority, either directly or via a 'subcon-
  tracting' arrangement for 'shared care' with a specialist provider
  unit. However, arrangements for this sort of reimbursement are
  poorly developed in most districts.

• Primary care teams who take sexual health promotion seriously
  may gain insights into patients' needs and preferences for
  specialist HIV/AIDS and GUM services, which can be used to
  advise health authorities on commissioning. In using their influence, however, GPs need to recognize that the patients they
  see may be a selected subset of those needing HIV/AIDS and
  GUM services. Health authorities should consider the needs of
  all patients, including those who find it difficult to use general
  practice services or are unwilling to do so.

• Specialist HIV/AIDS and GUM services do not fall within the
  established fund-holding scheme.

• With the introduction of pilot 'total fund-holding' projects,
  specialist GUM and HIV/AIDS providers are very concerned that
  the principle of open access to their services could be eroded.

9

Providing condoms

In response to 1992 Department of Health guidance encouraging district health authorities to consider supplying condoms to GPs, and to interest and pressure from primary care teams, there have been a number of schemes for distributing condoms in general practice. Most have been small-scale pilot schemes with five or six general practices participating for about six months. Following evaluation, some projects have ended, a few have been extended and several have expanded to make condoms available to all interested practices in the area. However, outside these schemes, there is no nationwide arrangement for general practices to obtain condoms for distribution to patients, and condoms are not a reimbursable item of practice expenditure. This section uses the lessons learned from the various evaluations to provide pointers for primary care teams considering whether or not to seek funding to distribute condoms.

What do heterosexual people think of condoms?

Condom promotion is the major thrust of global AIDS prevention programmes, as condoms are the only products that offer protection against both pregnancy and infections. However, research suggests that condom use is low among heterosexuals, and consistent use has not become integrated into people's lives.

- Large proportions of sexually active people aged 16–24 do not use condoms regularly.

- Condom use declines with increasing age.

- Condoms are not the preferred contraceptive option among couples who consider themselves to be in a steady or faithful relationship.

- Those who first have intercourse at the earliest age and those who have most partners are least likely to use condoms.

Research suggests the following possible reasons.

- There may be embarrassment about buying condoms, especially among the young, and a fear of being seen by someone one knows. Although most people feel that it should be acceptable for everyone to carry condoms, embarrassment and negative perceptions persist.

- There are real and perceived drawbacks, including lack of sexual spontaneity, reduced sensitivity for the male, aesthetic objections and reservations about efficacy.

- It is unclear to what extent negative attitudes to condoms among women are genuine as opposed to an internalization of their partners' views. Most young heterosexual women are more worried about pregnancy than HIV, and this may have a bearing on their views.

- There is some evidence that people have anchored their understanding of the new idea of HIV prevention in their pre-existing views of condoms as a method of contraception – suitable at the start of a relationship, but to be superseded by the pill as the relationship becomes established. This is problematic for HIV prevention, since there may be an on-going risk if the partner is infected through a previous or concurrent relationship.

- There is a need for a high level of motivation, since the condom has to be put on immediately prior to penetration. This may be adversely affected by alcohol or drugs.

The pilot schemes mentioned above shared a common basic structure but varied in detail.

- Most schemes offered training to support staff in providing condoms.

- Some used a predetermined protocol for condom distribution, while others were less directive and facilitated practice staff in developing their own protocols.

- Some schemes targeted particular groups of patients (e.g. young people or gay men) or specific consultations, while others offered condoms opportunistically to all patients.

- Several schemes distributed condom 'starter packs' as a way to encourage condom use and to create a context in which to discuss STDs and HIV, while a few aimed to give patients a regular supply of condoms.

Rationale for providing condoms

- To improve health in line with the *Health of the Nation* strategy

- Condom distribution provides an opportunity, and can be used as a tool, to raise awareness of STDs, HIV and sexual health

- Availability of condoms in general practice signals to patients that staff regard sexual health as important and are willing to discuss sexual health concerns

- Offering condoms reinforces sexual health information and advice

- Condoms provide an additional contraceptive choice within the accessible setting of general practice

- Providing condoms can benefit staff and deepen relationships with patients, by enabling a more holistic approach to health care and by providing an opportunity for professional development and confidence-building in a new area

---

Key questions that primary care teams should think about when considering condom distribution include the following.

What is the aim of providing condoms in our practice?

This needs to be clear, explicit and understood by all staff. Clear aims will suggest how the condom scheme should be organized (e.g. who will be offered condoms, how many, when and by whom?) and will assist in costing. Several questions about aims can be asked.

- Are condoms to be distributed primarily as a prophylactic against infections, as a method of contraception, or as both?

- Is the intention to supply patients with condoms for regular use over an extended period, or to provide a one-off intervention to raise awareness and encourage condom usage?

- Will condoms be given out by staff as part of a sexual health promotion package, or will condoms be accessible to patients to take for themselves?

Where can we get funding?

The ease of access to funds for condom distribution and actual condom supplies varies from area to area. It is likely to become harder as funding for HIV/AIDS work tightens up. In the first instance, practices could apply to the FHSA, health promotion unit or district HIV prevention co-ordinator for funding to distribute condoms. To stand a chance of success, it will probably be necessary to demonstrate a clear rationale and strategy, perhaps with a component of research and evaluation. It may also be possible to obtain condoms free or at a reduced cost from manufacturers for awareness-raising interventions, although not for regular supply. If funding is refused, the practice may consider less direct ways of promoting condom usage, such as:

- contacting local services that supply condoms to discuss ways of improving interagency referral. Free condoms are usually available from agencies such as family planning clinics, GUM clinics, young people's clinics and some drugs projects

- displaying posters on condom use and sexual health services in the waiting area and consultation rooms

- ensuring that a range of leaflets on condom use and sexual health services is available

- when discussing sexual health, talking about condom use and telling the patient where free condoms are available.

What organizational arrangements are needed?

The following practicalities should be addressed:

- financial and supply systems

- stock-check and order systems

- delivery of condoms

- appropriate storage conditions for condom supplies.

The local FHSA or health promotion department may be able to advise and assist in setting up workable arrangements.

How shall we publicize the availability of condoms?

Good publicity increases the number of patients who raise the issue of sexual health and condom use. Some staff may be concerned that active advertising of the service might offend patients, but evaluation of condom schemes shows this to be unjustified. Publicity may include:

- producing a poster on the service for display in the waiting area and consultation rooms

- a notice advertising the service in the practice leaflet

- exhibiting a display of condom leaflets and posters in the waiting area

- telling all patients, or new patients registering, that the practice supplies condoms.

Which patients will be offered condoms?

This should be decided in the light of the aims of the scheme and available resources. It could be all patients, specific patient groups or patients attending specific consultations and clinics.

If specific patient groups are to be targeted, criteria (e.g. age, sex, sexual preference and number of partners) need to be identified. The chosen criteria must be ones that can actually be applied. For example, if the criterion for offering condoms is a patient's sexual preference, staff need to know this and must therefore take appropriate sexual histories. Any targeting criteria should be decided in the light of available resources, the distribution aim, the reality of the working environment and the limits it imposes, and staff time, skills, knowledge and confidence. Written criteria help to ensure a consistent delivery of service, prompt staff to raise the issue with patients and provide legitimization and support for staff.

In which consultations will condoms be offered?

The following consultations have been identified by primary health care staff and patients as being the main situations in which it is appropriate to offer condoms:

•   general check-up or Well Woman/Man clinic

•   contraceptive consultation or clinic

•   new patient screening

•   travel vaccination clinics

•   pregnancy testing and postnatal care

•   smear testing

•   consultations about possible STDs.

The evaluations of condom schemes with a primary focus on HIV prevention have consistently shown that most condoms have been given to women (72–90%), aged 21–30 years old, and for the purpose of contraception (56–88%). This suggests that staff find it easiest to raise condom use in the context of contraceptive consultations with women. Ways of overcoming this may need to be sought if the aim of providing condoms is prophylaxis against infections. If one wishes to target patients who do not attend contraceptive consultations, for example gay men or heterosexual men, how can they be reached?

How will condoms be offered?

- They can be left in a basket in the waiting room or a private area (e.g. the toilet) for patients to pick up.
- Receptionists can participate in the distribution.
- Condoms can be given by clinical staff during consultations.
- Publicity can be displayed to tell patients condoms are available and invite them to ask staff for further information.

How many condoms and of what type shall we give?

If the aim is to promote condom use, rather than to provide a long-term supply, starter packs (providing a small selection of condoms) can be offered. However, if the aim is to provide an ongoing supply, it may be useful to decide upon a standard number and range of condoms to offer. Many professionals find it difficult to decide what type and number of condoms to offer to an individual patient, since this may require discussion of detailed sexual behaviour. A written protocol on the number and range of condoms to offer provides a framework for discussion and decision-making. It can be based on the number and range offered by the local family planning service.

The range of condoms stocked may also be influenced by the specific groups being targeted: for example, schemes aimed at young people often stock coloured and flavoured condoms. If more than one type is stocked, staff should be aware of the differences between them and be able to discuss this with patients, to assist them in choosing the most appropriate condom. The leaflet *Which condom?*[17] is a source of information.

Shall we give any information with the condoms?

Condom distribution can be used as an opportunity to give sexual health information in a number of ways: written leaflets, discussion and, where appropriate, a demonstration of condom use. Information can be standardized or tailored to individual patients to encourage them to raise any concerns they may have. Standardized information is quick, so can be given to a large number of people, but it may be difficult for people to use if it has little relevance to the individual. Tailored information is usually more time-consuming but may be more effective, as it can address the reality of the patient's situation.

Teaching correct condom use

Many people have misconceptions about how to use condoms. It is important to be able to give accurate instruction, with demonstration where possible. People who have not used condoms before may like to familiarize themselves with how to handle one before using one for intercourse.

1   Check that the packet carries a British Standards kitemark and that the 'use by' date has not been passed. In future, the kitemark may be superseded by an EU quality standard.

2   Immediately before use, open the wrapper of the individual condom carefully, avoiding tearing of the condom with fingernails, teeth, jewellery etc.

3   By rolling the rim of the condom gently between thumb and finger, one can feel how it will unroll, i.e. which is the inside and outside of the condom. However, do not unroll the condom before placing it over the penis.

4   Place the condom on the erect penis before penetration:

  •   squeeze the end of the condom to provide a small space for expansion and ejaculation

  •   then place it over the end of the penis, the right way out, and unroll it right down to the base of the penis.

5   After ejaculation, withdraw before the erection is lost, while carefully holding the condom around the base of the penis so that it does not slip off.

6   Used condoms can be disposed of by wrapping in tissue and throwing in the bin.

7   Use a new condom every time you have intercourse.

8   If a lubricant is used (essential for anal sex), it must be water-based. Vaseline, oils, hand lotions, moisturizers etc. damage

condoms and must be avoided. A little lubricant inside the tip of the condom enhances sensitivity for some men.

9 If using condoms for contraception, seek emergency contraception in the event of condom failure or non-use.

10 Be prepared to try different condom brands. You may find one you prefer.

Shall we record any information?

Condom distribution may raise concerns about the recording of information and confidentiality. It may be useful to consider these issues at a planning stage. For example, should discussion of a patient's sexuality or sexual relationship(s) be recorded in his or her notes?

- If yes, how will the information be used, how will it be recorded, who will have access to it and could it have any detrimental effect in the future?
- If no, how will staff use, remember or pass on any relevant information?

Framework for the development of a condom distribution protocol

- Project aim(s)
- Project objective(s)
- Publicity strategy
- Target population(s)
- Who will distribute the condoms?
- When will they be given (in what context)?

- What information will be given when condoms are offered?
- What issues will be raised when condoms are distributed?
- What range of condoms will be offered?
- How many condoms will be offered?
- How will information be recorded?
- How will distribution be monitored and evaluated?
- Timescale and costing for the proposal

10

Audit and evaluation

Professionals often perceive monitoring and evaluation of their work as time-consuming and of little use, and in some instances this may be true – especially where it is externally imposed. However, if applied effectively, monitoring and evaluation can have a direct impact on all levels of service provision, within the general practice itself and through the commissioning process. The benefits include:

- providing information on patient sexual health and existing services for use in commissioning

- assisting strategic planning and effective allocation of resources, at all levels (e.g. condom provision)

- providing qualitative information on professionals' and patients' views, to enable the improvement and development of service provision

- establishing a baseline of current practice by which to evaluate change

- identifying service difficulties and needs, and ways to address these

- offering a framework to facilitate and support change.

To date, monitoring and evaluation of sexual health services in general practice appears to have received little attention, and where examples do exist, they have mostly been commissioned by FHSAs or health promotion agencies and conducted by researchers external to general practice. However, the audit model whereby clinicians assess and appraise their own performance should provide a good framework for monitoring and evaluating sexual health promotion in general practice. By participating actively in planning of monitoring and evaluation, primary care teams may be able to ensure that the process takes account of the reality and limitations of their working environments, and that the results are disseminated in a manner that

The audit cycle

1 *Select* a service or an aspect of service to explore. The aim of the audit needs to be clearly defined, located within the service and realistic.

2 *Assess* existing practice. The aspects of current activity assessed need to be relevant to the aim of the audit and possible (given the likely restraints of time and resources) to collect and analyse.

3 *Set* clear service standards to achieve. Targets need to be identified in the light of available staff skills and resources.

4 *Identify* any discrepancies between the existing level of practice and the desired standard level.

5 *Clarify* what interventions and actions are required to bring the service up to the desired level. A range of interventions may be identified, for example staff training or protocol development.

6 *Implement* the required changes.

7 *Review* the service after an agreed period. On the basis of the review, standards can be refined and follow-up dates set for further review.

is useful to them in improving their service to patients. One example of an audit initiative is a proposal produced by Camden and Islington medical audit advisory group, in London, to raise awareness of issues associated with unplanned pregnancy and to improve provision of contraception in general practices. The objectives of this are:

• to document family planning services provided by general practice in the area

• to identify aspects of these services that may affect uptake and contribute to the local rate of termination of pregnancy

• to instigate educational opportunities about audit and contraception in primary care in order to raise awareness of the benefits of audit

- to facilitate changes to improve services, and to monitor the effects of those changes.

Examples of ways of reviewing and auditing contraceptive care

Although it is not possible to establish what the optimum uptake of contraception would be for a practice population, the proportion to whom a service is offered is an important baseline to inform subsequent work. It can be estimated by using the practice's age/sex register or FHSA database to determine the number of women of fertile age registered, and the proportion for whom claims for contraceptive payments are made, bearing in mind that some women will not need contraception because they are sexually inactive, lesbian, pregnant or trying to become so, or because they or their partner have been sterilized.

PACT data for prescriptions of oral contraceptives, spermicides and intrauterine devices can also be very informative. Discussion within the practice about the reasons for using different oral contraceptives can lead to establishment of a sensible shared 'formulary' and the most rational prescribing.

Other audit questions might cover:

- the types of contraception used by patients registered at the practice

- the proportion of women choosing various methods

- the methods of contraception used by women requiring pregnancy tests

- the last method used by women seeking termination of pregnancy

- referrals to STD clinics

- ways for patients registered at the practice to obtain methods of contraception that the practice does not provide (e.g. condoms, IUCDs, Norplant, diaphragms and Depo-Provera).

The method will involve a questionnaire to GPs, inviting them to choose areas for audit from the options:

- establishing a register for contraception

- contraceptive provision and staff training

- understanding contraceptive methods

- emergency contraception

- care of ethnic minorities

- patient satisfaction

- post-termination of pregnancy or postpartum contraception and care

- condoms

- record-keeping and FP1001s

- post-pregnancy testing contraception and care.

Once practices have been recruited and have chosen areas for audit, they will be visited by the audit facilitator and workshops will take place, prior to data collection, analysis, follow-up and dissemination of results through the participating practices.

Other possible audit topics might include:

- *a review of the level of knowledge of patients using oral contraceptives*, for example a study to establish patients' knowledge of the effectiveness of the pill after sickness and diarrhoea. This could involve a questionnaire administered to all patients attending the practice for contraceptive provision, and the information could be used to improve advice given to patients

- *an audit of practice nurse care of patients receiving oral contraceptives.* For example, are patients offered written information, and are blood pressure checks carried out regularly? This could be done by analysis of patient records

- audit and evaluation of *condom distribution* schemes (see above), cervical cytology and sexual history-taking.

Sources of data for clinical audit

There are various ways of obtaining data for clinical audit. The method chosen needs to be matched to the aims of the audit and the staff skills, time and resources available. Quantitative and qualitative methods can be combined or used to answer different types of question – typically *what* and *how many* for quantitative measures, while qualitative methods answer *why* and can be used to illustrate and interpret.

Analysis of patient records and notes can be used to review practice and service provision. For example, how many patients have sexual history information recorded and how many are receiving contraceptive services.

Financial claim returns (e.g. FP1001, FP1002 and FP1003) can be collated and analysed to give basic statistical information.

Questionnaires can use open or closed questions, or a combination of both, to get a mixture of quantitative and qualitative information. They can be administered face to face or by telephone, or can be designed for self-completion and distributed via the receptionist, other staff or post.

Proformas (e.g. using a system of tick boxes) can be designed for staff to monitor particular aspects of their practice, for example when and how they give out leaflets and condoms.

Focus groups are facilitated groups of people who are invited to discuss their views and experience on a specific issue. They can be used to gain information from people such as patients using a particular service, GPs, practice nurses, referral services, commissioners and purchasers.

Interviews can take several forms, categorized by the level of planned structure imposed by the interviewer: in depth, semi-structured or structured.

Observation and participant observation, whereby information is gained by systematically recording observations in a particular setting or situation. In participant observation, the observer takes part in the process which he or she is observing.

11

Professional development, counselling approaches to health promotion and motivational skills

This section may be of particular relevance to GPs and practice nurses who are interested in counselling and psychotherapeutic approaches to primary care. It explores some of the underlying ideas behind sexual health promotion methods. It is based on the experience of the National AIDS Counselling Training Unit, a unit funded by the Department of Health, which offers PGEA-accredited training for GPs as well as courses for other NHS professionals.

The *Health of the Nation* challenges health professionals to work to reduce unplanned pregnancy and sexually transmitted disease, but has also triggered exploration of the meaning of sexual health and whether it fits within the existing framework, which is largely predicated on contraception, disease control and the treatment of dysfunction. For example, the World Health Organization definition of sexual health requires a number of components to come together for a person to be considered sexually healthy. He or she needs:

- a capacity to enjoy and control sexual and reproductive behaviour in accordance with a social and personal ethic

- freedom from fear, shame, guilt, false beliefs and other psychological factors inhibiting sexual response and impairing sexual relationships

- freedom from organic disorders, diseases and deficiencies that interfere with sexual and reproductive functions.

This helps to define the potential breadth of sexual health promotion, yet each of the above components raises issues that have a direct bearing on service delivery and on the training of health professionals.

Considering the first point, how does an individual define a *'personal and social ethic'*? Can there ever be an absolute code shared by all? Collectively and individually, how do we manage the range of ethnic, cultural and religious ethics currently operating in our society? Individually, how do we cope with changes in personal ethic or the fact that our principles and practices may be at odds with social norms?

Secondly, how do individuals free themselves from *fear and shame* about sexual identities and practices in a culture that is essentially 'sex negative'? How does this negativity affect people outside the mainstream, for example those who enjoy sex with others of the same sex? How do societal values affect the psychological well-being of those who do not conform? Research suggests a link between poor mental health in gay men and internalized negative images of homosexuality. How might responses to the sexual health needs of patients be undermined by professional discomfort, homophobia and sexism within the teams in which we work?

Lastly, *freedom from organic disorders* appears at first sight to be straightforward and within the remit of conventional health care. Where, however, does it leave people whose 'organic disorders' cannot be remedied? People with physical disabilities or learning difficulties may have normal sexual function but may be desexualized by preconceptions that healthy sex equates with healthy bodies. How do we respond to people whom we consider to have 'disorders' that they have 'chosen' or had imposed by cultural forces, for example circumcised or infibulated women?

Aspects of professional competence in sexual health

To work successfully in this broader conception of sexual health, professionals need training that addresses three essential areas: knowledge, values and skills. These represent the key building blocks for the development of the 'sexual health-aware worker'.

Knowledge

This refers not only to symptomatology, diagnosis and treatment, but also to the knowledge of different identities and practices, and the sociocultural dynamics surrounding them. Beyond this, the professional needs a working knowledge of disciplines to which he or she might refer, for example psychosexual medicine.

Exploring values

The second key building block refers to the professional exploring his or her beliefs, attitudes and values about a range of sexual practices and identities, and taking some responsibility for the effect these may have on the patient–practitioner relationship. Sexual health promotion is never a purely scientific, objective discipline, but is influenced by belief systems and how these are processed by individual practitioners. Professionals may sometimes be confronted with an individual whose sexual identity, practices or experiences challenge their own beliefs so profoundly that it is difficult to care for the person effectively.

However, good service delivery depends on an environment of trust in which patients feel free to disclose all relevant details of their sexual history. A brusque or unsupportive reaction from a professional is likely to compound the person's difficulties in relation to sexual identity or practice, and consequently psychosexual health, as well as deterring him or her from using the service in future.

It is thus the professional's responsibility to *enable* the patient to be honest. This can be difficult, since inner feelings of embarrassment or fear of being judged may sensitize patients to unconscious manifestations of discomfort, such as body language and tone of voice, on the part of the professional. The primary health care setting offers both pros and cons: on the one hand, the patient–professional relationship can be developed over time, but on the other hand there may be difficult issues where, say, a GP is treating several members of a family and managing confidential information about under-age sexual activity.

Acquiring skills

While clinical skills reflect different professional disciplines and remits, all workers need communication and interpersonal skills to foster a productive relationship with clients. An important aspect is to mediate and find a balance between the *task* component of the relationship (i.e. the aim to be achieved) and *maintenance* of the relationship itself, which involves interpersonal and emotional dynamics, such as embarrassment, fear of retribution and anxieties about confidentiality. (These terms are taken from the theory of experiential group work.)

For example, the task component might be to take a sexual history, and the maintenance component may be to pay attention to the emotional dynamics involved and create a safe environment. At the same time, each individual will have an inner landscape of needs, hopes and fears. Where equal attention is paid to the task, maintenance and personal needs dimensions of the consultation, and the needs of the patient do not clash with those of the worker, the encounter is likely to be productive. Both parties have their needs met, and the task can be accomplished within a climate in which the patient feels safe and is enabled to be honest.

Health promotion methods

In parallel with the concept of sexual health, that of health promotion raises difficult issues. The assumption is that health professionals should work to change the behaviour of their patients, but this is not straightforward. Can we change our patients? Should we change our patients? How do we change our patients? In practice, it is often difficult to change patients' behaviour.

Health workers are used to talking to patients about smoking, drinking and diet. Consultations commonly include the giving of advice and information, controlled by the worker. Giving advice works with some patients, and providing information may assist the decision-making process, but success rates are not high. How can health professionals negotiate change with patients, rather than simply persuade them to change?

Changing sexual behaviour is a particular challenge, since patients resist change being advocated on the basis of knowledge, attitudes or beliefs that they do not share. Patients attending with an STD or sexual health problem may show a high level of concern and stated desire to change. However, it is often not their behaviour so much as the infection that they wish to change. Once the STD has been treated, the concern may evaporate. At best, many patients are highly ambivalent about changing their behaviour. The professional's agenda also needs to be identified: does he or she have an implicit view of the desirability of change, or a willingness to work with the patient's notion of change and/or its desirability?

A helpful model of change

This model has been developed by analysis of smokers trying to give up. It identifies a six-stage cycle through which any person considering change will to some degree travel, sometimes several times:

- precontemplation of change

- contemplation

- decision to change – if this is not implemented, the person may return to precontemplation

- action – changing

- maintaining the changed behaviour

- relapsing to the previous behaviour – from where the cycle can start again.

The cycle is a powerful tool for assessing how to work with patients. Professionals often base interventions on an assumption that people are in the more advanced stages of action, or at least decision – 'they came here; they must want to do something about it'.

However, in reality, patients are often in the earlier stages of precontemplation or contemplation and show ambivalence, for example the 'Yes, but...' syndrome. If this ambivalence is not explored, it is hardly surprising that the desire for change evaporates once the person's immediate concern (e.g. a treatable STD) has been dealt with.

Ambivalence lies at the root of the change process and should be the focus of intervention. Professionals who want to develop their health promotion skills might wish to seek training in motivational interviewing, a client-centred technique for examining ambivalence and helping people to change without persuasion or coercion. It is particularly helpful for clients in the (pre)contemplative stage. In motivational interviewing, the professional seeks to assist the client's internal process of change, reinforcing the client's competence and belief that he or she best knows what changes to make and how. The worker presents selective arguments for not changing, based on the client's stage in the cycle of change, while the client presents arguments for change. This makes use of the discrepancy between what the patient is doing and what he or she may want to do or be. The worker's role is to draw out and work with the key elements of conflict the patient feels between his or her present behaviour and future goals, to examine the costs and benefits both of changing and of staying the same. Further strategies, for *how* to change, are not explored until ambivalence about the decision to change has been resolved.

Ambivalence is normal and common, but how health professionals respond to it is crucial. If the professional falls into the trap of taking responsibility for the reasons for change, the client is left to defend the reasons against. With the appropriate skills, the professional can assist the client in working through ambivalence and, where necessary, can then provide additional skills and strategies for change.

Practitioners who wish to develop a counselling-based approach to in-depth sexual health promotion need to acquire:

- sound clinical knowledge of sex-related disorders and their treatment

- a sound working knowledge of relevant law and ethical guidelines

- a good knowledge of relevant referral services and procedures

- a developed self-awareness relating to a broad range of sexual identities and practices

- knowledge of 'difficult' areas for him or her personally, and strategies for preventing these from interfering with the development of productive relationships with patients

- a range of interpersonal and communication skills to facilitate a climate of trust when assessing individuals' sexual health needs

- an awareness of personal and attitudinal limitations and when to refer on patients whose needs can be better met elsewhere.

Tutors and trainers supporting such practitioners would need to:

- explore and use experiential teaching methods to develop these competencies

- assess their skills in using non-didactic approaches and obtain appropriate training, for example based on National AIDS Counselling Training Unit principles of experiential teaching for sexual health education

- work to identify measurable skills and competencies for sexual health professionals.

GPs committed to developing and improving sexual health among patients could seek to:

- address the practice's overall response to sexuality and sexual health

- develop practice protocols on clinical and attitudinal aspects of sexual health work

- create contexts in which staff can air concerns and diffi-culties in relation to sexual health service delivery, and which recognize and accommodate diverse personal values, vul-nerabilities and belief systems.

Training and professional development

GPs and nurses who wish to acquire the sorts of skills discussed above will have to commit themselves to an exploration of self that is not always easy. Training should use experiential methods to re-cognize each individual's unique experience of sex and sexuality, and of strategies for working with it, and consequently their unique

contribution to the learning process. By allowing students to experience the concepts of task, maintenance and personal needs directly
as participants in an experiential group, they quickly develop the
awareness and skills to manage these dynamics in the work setting.
Further work is needed in defining the skills and competencies
needed for successful work in sexual health, and how these can be
measured and validated within academic frameworks.

References and further reading

References

1 Hoolaghan T, Blache G and Pidcock J (1993) *The role of general practitioners in HIV prevention: findings from a questionnaire survey.* The Health Promotion in General Practice Project. Camden and Islington Health Promotion Service, London.

2 Health Education Authority–BMA Foundation for AIDS Consultation Project (1993) Unpublished background paper and report of interviews. HEA/BMA, London.

3 Bond S, Rhodes TJ, Philips PR, Setters JK, Foy CJW and Bond J (1988) A national study of HIV infection, AIDS and community nursing staff in England. Health Care Research Unit, Report No. 35, University of Newcastle upon Tyne, Newcastle. (Out of print.)

4 Jewitt C (1993) *Towards effective HIV prevention and condom distribution in general practice. A research study in general practice.* Kensington & Chelsea and Westminster Commissioning Agency, London.

5 Weston A (1993) Challenging assumptions. *Nursing Times.* **89**: 26–7.

6 Schering Health Care Ltd (1993) *Contraception and sex in 1993.* Schering Health Care Ltd, Burgess Hill.

7 In 1990–91, 18.7% of women and 27.6% of men aged 16–19 at the time of interview said that they had had heterosexual intercourse before they reached the age of 16. Wellings K, Field J, Johnson AM and Wadsworth J (1994) *Sexual behaviour in Britain: the national survey of sexual attitudes and lifestyles.* Penguin, London.

8 Gallagher M *et al.* (1990) HIV and AIDS in England and Wales: general practitioners' workload and contact with patients. *British Journal of General Practice.* **40**: 154–7.

9 North West Thames Regional Health Authority (1989) *Making family planning services more HIV aware: a training pack for HIV prevention.* North West Thames Regional Health Authority HIV Project. London.

10 Brown-Peterside P, Sibbald B and Freeling P (1991) AIDS: knowledge, skills and attitudes among vocational trainees and their trainers. *British Journal of General Practice.* **41**: 401–5.

11 Fitzpatrick R, Dawson J, Boulton M *et al.* (1994) Perceptions of general practice among homosexual men. *British Journal of General Practice.* **44**: 80–2.

12 King E, Rooney M and Scott P (1992) *HIV prevention for gay men: a survey of initiatives in the UK.* North West Thames Regional Health Authority, London.

13 Zera D (1992) Coming of age in a heterosexist world: the development of gay and lesbian adolescents. *Adolescence.* **27**: 849–54.

14 Unlinked anonymous HIV prevalence monitoring programme in England and Wales: data to the end of 1993. Report from the Unlinked Anonymous HIV Surveys Steering Group. Department of Health, London.

15 Weatherburn P, Hunt AJ, Hickson FCI and Davies PM (1992) *The sexual lifestyles of gay and bisexual men in England and Wales.* Project Sigma, London.

16 Davies PM, Hickson FCI, Weatherburn P and Hunt AJ (1993) *Sex, gay men and AIDS.* Falmer Press, London.

17 *Which condom?* (leaflet showing different shapes and types available, currently in its third edition). Available from City and Hackney Young People's Project, St Leonards Hospital, London N1 5LZ.

Further reading

Adler M (1990) *ABC of sexually transmitted diseases,* 2nd edn. BMJ Publishing Group, London.

Adler M (ed.) (1993) *ABC of AIDS,* 3rd edn. BMJ Publishing Group, London.

Annon JS (1976) The PLISSIT model: a proposed conceptual scheme for the behavioural treatment of sexual problems. *Journal of Sex Education Therapists.* **2**: 1–15.

Armstrong EM and Gordon P (1992) *Sexualities: an advanced training resource.* Family Planning Association, London.

Belfield T (1993) *FPA contraceptive handbook: the essential reference guide for family planning and other health professionals.* Family Planning Association, London.

British Medical Association (1994) *Confidentiality and people under 16: guidance issued jointly by the BMA, GMSC, HEA, Brook Advisory Centres, FPA and RCGP* (free leaflet). BMA, London.

British Medical Association Foundation for AIDS (1992) *HIV infection and AIDS: ethical considerations for the medical profession,* 2nd edn. (booklet, single copies free). BMA Foundation for AIDS, London.

Brook Advisory Centres (1994) *Private and confidential: talking to doctors* (leaflet for young people, produced jointly by the BMA, GMSC, Brook Advisory Centres, FPA and RCGP). Brook Advisory Centres, London.

Cross E (1993) *The more you talk about it, the easier it gets...evaluation of the Sheffield condom pilot project* (research report). Sheffield FHSA and Sheffield Centre for HIV and Sexual Health, Sheffield.

Curtis H (ed.) (1992) *Promoting sexual health* (proceedings of the second international workshop on the prevention of sexual transmission of HIV and other STDs). BMA Foundation for AIDS, London.

Department of Health (1991) *Drug misuse and dependence: guidelines on clinical management.* HMSO, London.

Department of Health (1993) *Health of the Nation key area handbook: HIV/AIDS and sexual health.* HMSO, London.

Department of Health (1994) *HIV and AIDS – issues in primary care* (training pack). Department of Health, London.

English National Board for Nursing, Midwifery and Health Visiting (1994) *Caring for people with sexually transmitted diseases including HIV disease* (open learning pack). ENB, London.

English National Board for Nursing, Midwifery and Health Visiting (1994) *Sexual health education and training – guidelines for good practice* (booklet). ENB, London.

Family Planning Association (1995) *Your guide to contraception* (leaflet, compares different contraceptive methods). FPA, London.

Gordon P and Mitchell L (1988) *Safer sex – a new look at sexual pleasure.* Faber and Faber, London.

Green R (ed.) (1975) *Human sexuality: a health practitioner's text.* Waverley Press, Baltimore.

Health Education Authority (1992) *Chlamydia and NSU: What they are and what you can do about them* (booklet). HEA, London.

Health Education Authority (1992) *Genital warts: what they are and what to do about them* (booklet). HEA, London.

Health Education Authority (1992) *Gonorrhoea: what it is and what to do about it* (booklet). HEA, London.

Health Education Authority (1992) *Vaginal infections: what they are and what to do about them* (booklet). HEA, London.

Health Education Authority (1994) *Health update 4: sexual health* (booklet summarizing health statistics and recent research results). HEA, London.

Ingram-Fogel C and Lauver D (1990) *Sexual health promotion* (includes discussion of the effects on sexual functioning of certain drugs, medical conditions and surgical procedures). WB Saunders, Philadelphia.

International Planned Parenthood Federation (1992) *Counselling and sexuality: a video-based training resource* (4 videos and manual). Hygia Communications, London.

Jewitt C (1995) *Sexual history taking in general practice* (research report). The HIV Project, London.

Mansfield S and Singh S (1990) *The management of HIV infection in primary care* (booklet). BMA Foundation for AIDS, London.

National AIDS manual – AIDS Directory (1994) (directory of services). NAM Publications, London.

Pengilley L and Kay R (1992) *Letters – french and free* (research report). Oxfordshire FHSA and DHA, Oxford.

Royal College of General Practitioners (1991) *Family planning and sexual health: a policy statement on clinical service provision.* RCGP, London.

Somerset Health Authority (1993) *Evaluation of GP condom scheme* (research report). Somerset Health Authority, Taunton.

Wellings K, Field J, Johnson A and Wadsworth J (1994) *Sexual behaviour in Britain – the national survey of sexual attitudes and lifestyles.* Penguin, London.

West London Health Promotion Agency (1993) *The Hillingdon GP condom project – an evaluation* (research report). West London Health Promotion Agency, Southall, London.

Worrall J and Aylesbury C (1992) *General practice condom and sexual health promotion trial* (research report). Derbyshire Family Health Services Authority, Derby.

Useful addresses

Advice, resources and materials such as leaflets and posters should be available from FHSAs and local health promotion departments, but the following sources may also be helpful for information, training and advice:

Age Concern (has produced a video 'Living, loving and ageing', about elderly people's sexual health)
Astrol House
1268 London Road
London   SW16 4ER
Tel: 0181 679 8000

AIDS Help Line – Northern Ireland
310 Bryson House
Bedford Street
Belfast   BT2 7FE
Tel: (01232) 249268

Association to Aid the Sexual and Personal Relationships of People with a Disability (SPOD)
286 Camden Road
London   N7 0BJ
Tel: 0171 607 8851

Black HIV/AIDS Network (BHAN)
Main Office: St Stephen's House
41 Uxbridge Road
London   W12 8LH
Tel: 0181 749 2828
Fax: 0181 746 2898

Body Positive
51b Philbeach Gardens
Earls Court
London   SW5 9EB
Tel: 0171 835 1045
Tel: 0171 373 9124 Helpline (Mon–Fri 7 pm–10pm, Sat–Sun
4 pm–10 pm)

British Medical Association Foundation for AIDS
BMA House
London   WC1H 9JP
Tel: 0171 383 6345/6315
Fax: 0171 388 2544

Brook Advisory Centres
Education and Publications Unit
165 Grays Inn Road
London   WC1X 8UD
Tel: 0171 833 8488
Fax: 0171 833 8182

Communicable Diseases Surveillance Centre
Central Public Health Laboratory
61 Colindale Avenue
London   NW9 5HT
Tel: 0181 200 4400

Department of Health AIDS Unit
Friars House
157/168 Blackfriars Road
London   SE1 8EU
Tel: 0171 972 2000

The Durex Information Service for Sexual Health
c/o Stuart Dimaline
LRC Products Ltd
North Circular Road
London   E4 8QA
Tel: 0181 527 2377
Fax: 0181 503 3100

Family Planning Association
27/35 Mortimer Street
London W1N 7RJ
Tel: 0171 636 7866 or 0171 631 0555
Fax: 0171 436 3288

General Medical Council
178–202 Great Portland Street
London W1N 6JE
Tel: 0171 580 7642

Haemophilia Society
123 Westminster Bridge Road
London SE1 7HR
Tel: 0171 928 2020
Fax: 0171 620 1416

Health Education Authority
Hamilton House
Mabledon Place
London WC1H 9TX
Tel: 0171 383 3833
Fax: 0171 387 0550

Health Promotion Authority for Wales
8th Floor
Brunel House
2 Fitzalan Road
Cardiff CF2 1EB
Tel: (01222) 472472

The Institute of Psychosexual Medicine
11 Chandos Street
London W1M 9DE
Tel: 0171 580 0631

London Lighthouse
111/117 Lancaster Road
London W11 1QT
Tel: 0171 792 1200
Fax: 0171 964 2543

Mainliners
205 Stockwell Road
London   SW9 9SL
Tel: 0171 737 7472
Tel: 0171 737 3141 (Helpline)
Fax: 0171 737 3361

National AIDS Counselling Training Units (NACTU)
NACTU (London)
St Charles' Hospital
Exmoor Street
London   W10 6DZ
Tel: 0181 968 8514
Fax: 0181 960 9915

National AIDS Help line
PO Box LB400
London   WC2B 6JG
0800 567123 (Freephone)

Positively Women
5 Sebastian Street
London   EC1V 0HE
Tel: 0171 490 5501 (Office)
Tel: 0171 490 2327 (Helpline)

Relate
Herbert Gray College
Little Church Street
Rugby
Warwickshire   CV21 3AP
Tel: (01788) 573241

Royal College of Nursing (RCN)
HIV Nursing Society
c/o RCN
20 Cavendish Square
London   W1M 0AB
Tel: 0171 409 3333
Fax: 0171 495 6104 (mark 'HIV Nursing Society')

Scottish AIDS Monitor
PO Box 48
Edinburgh   EH1 3SA
Tel: 0131 557 3885

Scottish Health Education Group
Health Education Centre
Woodburn House
Canaan Lane
Edinburgh   EH10 4SG
Tel: 0131 447 8044

Scottish Home and Health Department
St Andrew House
Edinburgh   EH1 3DE
Tel: 0131 556 8400

Sexually Transmitted Disease
(STD) Clinic, Special or Genito-Urinary
See telephone directory under 'VD' or 'Venereal Disease'

Spinal Injuries Association
76 St James Lane
London   N10 3DA
Tel: 0181 444 2121

Standing Conference on Drug Abuse (SCODA)
1/4 Hatton Place
London   EC1N 8ND
Tel: 0171 928 9500
Fax: 0171 928 7071

Terrence Higgins Trust (THT)
52–54 Grays Inn Road
London   WC1X 8JU
Tel: 0171 831 0330 (Office)
Tel: 0171 242 1010 (Helpline)

Index